My Life as a Metal Sculpture:
Navigating through Medical Adversity

My Life as a Metal Sculpture:
Navigating Through Medical Adversity

CAROL R. PALO

LUMINARE PRESS

EUGENE, OREGON

My Life as a Metal Sculpture: Navigating through Medical Adversity
© 2013 Carol R. Palo

Printed in the United States of America

Cover Design: Claire Last
Spine Illustration: Emily Goetz

Luminare Press
467 W 17th Ave
Eugene, OR 97401
www.luminarepress.com

LCCN: 2013952298
ISBN: 978-1-937303-18-1

CONTENTS

Part One
My Story

Part Two
Perspectives

Part Three
Helpful Tools and Resources

INTRODUCTION

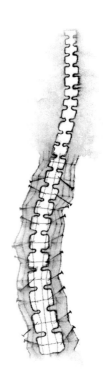

Beautiful titanium
Bone and protein mass
Nerves severed and reconnected
Abstract but functional art,
   relieving me of pain
   giving me the ability
   to live life anew
That is real beauty

My medical adversity involved a deteriorating spine that twisted, bent, and rotated, driving my rib cage into my pelvis. It was unexpected, unwanted, frightening.

Life sometimes hands us medical trauma, and by us, I mean not just those of us whose bodies are involved, but also loved ones, coworkers, and neighbors. All in our circle are affected.

Using my experience in getting through the trauma, I've written this book as a guide for anyone with these questions: What next? What do I do? How can good decisions be made? Do I have choices? What do I tell people? How do I move forward? What can I expect? I offer suggestions to help you attain emotional balance and hope, how to accept and identify the reality of what is going on.

My Life is divided into three parts. The first is a narrative about what I went through, starting with hearing about the severity of my problem. The journey and process of moving through disbelief, questions, decisions, and actions disclose how I was able to reclaim a fulfilling life.

The second is a reminder of the impact we have on those close to us, including comments and helpful tips from family and friends. Also included are stories from others who found themselves in precarious medical situations and what helped them.

The third contains lists, actions, forms, and resources. If you have no patience for reading my story, feel free to go directly to the resource section for ideas you can use immediately.

PART ONE
MY STORY

To live is so startling it leaves little time for anything else.
—Emily Dickenson

CHAPTER 1

WHAT IS HAPPENING TO ME?

~~⌒

*A*lthough I was very active and felt I was getting healthier not older, I began to wonder if I was getting arthritis in my back because pain and balance issues started to develop. I guessed the discomfort was a result of not doing enough of the right exercises.

One day I looked in the mirror and focused on my back. It was clearly out of kilter. I had a vague feeling something was really wrong, and it scared me. I didn't want to deal with the possibility, but I finally looked for orthopedic doctors in my insurance network and neighborhood and made an appointment. The doctor took X-rays, then stood with his back to me, running his fingers over the X-ray. I felt that awkward pause nobody wants to feel at the doctor's office. Why did he seem to be searching for words?

My head played that quick game of Oh, you're just nervous and imagining the space of time and lack of words. Maybe the doctor just has a dramatic flair or a slightly warped sense of humor. Most likely he is just going to chide you for not taking better care of yourself. After all, you're not a kid anymore. The body just naturally gets aches and pains.

But my first instinct was right, and the words that finally came weren't good.

I left his office and sat in my car for a long time, not even knowing what to do with the information I now had. I didn't know how I felt and didn't know what to do next. Then I felt a sense of surrealism and numbness followed by fear, anger, and the attempt to disclaim and disown both the present and the future.

What was I to do with the diverse but simultaneous desires to scream 'Unfair! Look at what is happening to me!' and 'Be very, very quiet, because if you don't tell anyone, it won't be happening.' Then came waves of shame and embarrassment (what have I done, what haven't I done), then the sobering realization of how it would impact everyone and everything in my life.

Well, that was my first forty-eight hours.

Today I am grateful for the brutal honesty of the specialist as he told me he wouldn't sugarcoat his prognosis or what I would need to do. When I was twelve years old I had been diagnosed with scoliosis (a spinal curvature). I did exercises for several years, which stabilized the situation. I gave it no more thought. I gave birth to two children without problems, worked, and traveled. In my forties I noticed that when I was tired, I had difficulty standing up straight. I seemed to lean to one side. In my mid-fifties I started having real problems with pain in my hips and back. I had been tested for osteoporosis and knew my bones were in good shape.

I didn't know that some inner spinal programming could activate the *Let's rotate and curve the spinal column until it pushes itself into the pelvis.* It happens to only a small percentage of scoliosis patients—and I was one of them. This, the X-rays showed, was the source of my pain and new clumsiness.

"It's physics," said the doctor. "As the rotation and curving continues, it will reach the point of no return and your rib cage will be pushed into your pelvis. Severe pain, debilitation, and loss of living, as you know it today, will follow." He added, "Of course, the body is full of surprises. It is possible that the rotation and downward spiral will inexplicably stop. And there is no way to know how long the process will really take until you are quite disabled. It could be a couple of years or it might take seven or eight years."

He paused, adding, "You can take a chance on the long odds that the progression will just stop before too much damage is done. You can stall a decision by trying exercise, back braces, physical therapy, and whatever else you find that relieves the pain. You could surrender to the inevitable outcome of needing extreme surgery. The surgery involves taking apart and rebuilding your spine and requires cutting all the nerves and later reattaching them in the area requiring rebuilding, in your case most of your spine. Double titanium rods and screws will be put in place, and bending will be only possible at the hip level. The only other recourse is to resign yourself to being in a wheelchair in a nursing home on medication and in pain as your new normal life in a few years."

Since I hadn't heard him offer any options I could imagine taking, I asked him what he would do. He said he'd take a chance on the extreme surgery, one so extreme he wouldn't perform it because the complication rate was very high and the surgery would best be performed by a doctor and team who regularly specialized in this type of surgery. He advised looking for a good track record of successful surgeries.

He asked me, "What kind of a life would you have without the surgery? Think of living in a nursing home, unable to walk, and in pain even with heavy medication. Would you be willing to settle for that?"

As I got ready to leave, he mentioned, "I plan to see a friend this evening who performs these extreme surgeries. I'll bring your X-rays along and see if he thinks you're a good candidate. Make an appointment to see me next week, and we can discuss what comes next. I told you, I'm not going to let you just go home and pretend this isn't happening."

I thought, He's taking my X-rays to a visit with his friend? Is this his dry sense of humor? Is he that dedicated? Is my back that bad?

I left the office completely stunned. I didn't know what to think or what to feel. The next day I went to work but was so nonfunctional I couldn't accomplish much. After a second night of little sleep, I decided I had better take a day off from work and somehow come to terms with what was to become of me. What could I do to make sense of the changes ahead and find direction?

For me, being out in nature has always been calming and usually makes me feel in balance with my life and the planet. I packed a beverage and bite to eat as well as a notebook and pen. As I wandered the paths of Portland's Japanese Garden, I knew I would have to put my thoughts and fears on paper. I would need to look at what was at my disposal in the way of assets and liabilities. I would need to come up with a plan.

Here's what I wrote:

POSITIVES

- I have time to decide about whether to have surgery or not.
- I have a friend who has a friend who avoided back surgery with some exercises. I could check into that.
- Other doctors might have more options.
- I can look at alternative medicine for solutions.
- It's not a fatal disease.
- I have a really good support base of family and friends available if I ask them to help me.

FEARS

- Will I be crippled and end up in chronic pain before I'm even ready to retire? It could happen to me in my early sixties.
- If I have surgery and the best surgeon resides out of town, the surgery might need to be in another city or state. How would that work? Would I lose my job? Would insurance pay? Where would I live? Who would help me?
- Who will look after my mom? (I'm an only child and my mom is in her nineties in assisted living. She always says, "What would

I do without you?" and I always answer, "Don't worry, I'll always be here to help you.")

GOOD IDEAS FROM A FEW CLOSE FRIENDS, MY SON, AND MY DAUGHTER (THE PEOPLE I CALLED IN THE FIRST TWENTY-FOUR HOURS AFTER THE DOCTOR VISIT)

- Get references from people who have had the surgery.
- Go to a back specialty shop; for example, get a zero gravity chair.
- Remember to pray; keep God in the loop, be directed.
- Call friends I trust for reality checks.
- Remember Thomas Edison's quote: "Loss of everything is also freedom for all new things."
- Use meditation to get answers from my body (even specifics like "How long do I have before my body is in too much pain, too crippled?").
- Breathe; get to a position of neutrality and ask to be open to what comes next or later.
- Remember to see the gifts that will come with the situation.
- Remember that whatever happens—surgery, debilitation—I'm still me and will still be loved.
- Separate out fears and emotional distress from what is really happening to my body, like structural changes and pains. That way I can deal with the truth of what is actually happening.
- Pray for clarity and the greater good.

POSITIVE RESOURCES

- A friend who survived cancer and changed her entire life style, a survivor with the courage to do whatever it takes to have quality of life.
- A chiropractor who also has a spiritual bent and alternative health resources.
- A boyfriend's promise of love and support.
- My two wonderful adult children who would stand by me and help me no matter what. What a fortunate thing it is if after

My Life as a Metal Sculpture 5

our children grow up a whole new relationship of being equals in friendship happens.

- A good friend at work who has been through great difficulty and is willing to share the experiences and solutions as well as a willingness to just listen when that's needed.
- A close friend who survived open-heart surgery followed by a heart attack as well as seeing his wife through cancer. He offers straight truths and has a spiritual program to live by.
- My spiritual sister, the coauthor of an unpublished book we have been working on for several years. She will be there for me.
- A friend in the Midwest who developed her own horrific back problems. Now comes the opportunity to share our fears, what to do next, how our lives will change.
- A friend I worked with years ago who had a similar back problem. The curvature was in her upper back. The surgery was not quite as severe as what I am facing, but it was successful. She would understand what I am going through.
- A doctor who will help me find a way to make the best decision I possibly can.

WHAT I WANT TO DO BEFORE I AM BADLY CRIPPLED OR HAVE SURGERY

- Take my family to see the Blue Man Group show in Las Vegas; in fact, take the family for a little vacation in Las Vegas, even if it's just one or two nights.
- Make love—lots.
- Exercise and experience lots of bending and flexing. Really pay attention to what my body can do and how it all feels while I still can.
- Travel, always my passion, around the world if possible.

THINGS THAT NEED TO BE DONE PRIOR TO SURGERY OR BEING TOO DISABLED TO WORK

- Check insurances and disability plan.
- Do my best work so I can be as sure as possible to keep my job.

- Do what I can to find out what it would be like either crippled or after the surgery for the following activities:
- Driving a car
- Having sex
- Walking up or down stairs
- Walking at all
- Pain management
- Make a real will and fill out an advance directives form.
- Regarding my mom, take appropriate action when the time comes to see that she is taken care of and will be told as much as she needs to know.

I drove a little farther to the Rose Garden, which overlooks the city. There were lots of benches to sit on while I ate lunch. It was a much-needed opportunity to enjoy the view, smell fragrant flowers, and just breathe before writing more.

What came to me in the midst of the fragrance, soft sculpted roses, and crystal clear sky was, to my surprise, a sense of gratitude and direction. I wrote:

Thank you God —
For all this beauty
For enough grace to turn this corner
For knowledge of your presence
For the opportunity to relax in your sunshine
    (literal and otherwise)
For right now, at least, that the fear moves to an outer ring on
    the bulls-eye of my new horizon.

Some random thoughts that first week
- Last couple of days I've felt sneezy, hot and cold, with a scratchy throat—like a cold or flu bug or maybe it's stress—a reaction to what's going on.

- Surgery concerns: I may be too old to handle up to twenty hours of anesthetic. I think about my mom's reaction after her last hip surgery. She never really was mentally sharp as before. (Yes, she is thirty-seven years older than I am, but still, she had that reaction.) Also, the doctor doesn't even know about my abnormal EEGs and the fragility of the bones in my neck from car accidents.
- When I talked to my chiropractor about the doctor's prognosis for my back, she told me of her sister who was diagnosed with MS two years ago and is having a hard time with it. She said, "It's interesting how our blessings are given to us, directions and people in ways we would never choose."
- Before God can give me direction to my consciousness, I feel I must ask for that assistance. But first my mind needs to be cleared to receive direction that will be more helpful than are my fears or emotions. I'm not sure how empty it needs to be, but certainly a lot of fear, anger, and wondering need to be released to make room.

I went back to the specialist. His friend who does these extreme surgeries had looked at my X-rays and thought I would be a good candidate. The specialist suggested I consult with several doctors who do these surgeries and gave me some questions I should ask and some things to look for. He provided me with the names and locations of three doctors, including his friend. I made an appointment with his friend first.

I went back to work and let myself be absorbed by all those things, people, and activities that normally fill my waking hours. Now it all seemed very finite instead of endlessly rolling out in front of me.

I made a list of questions I could use for all the doctor interviews and realized I was handling this like a business project, sort of like a request for proposals I might do when purchasing a large piece of

Carol R. Palo

equipment or new services. It seemed right that the business of what happens to my life would be as important to me as any work I might do for an employer.

These are the questions I determined to ask all the doctors and the information I thought they should have about me. The list is a combination of what my first doctor suggested I ask and questions that came to me that, it seemed, would help me make the most informed decision.

- What is your prognosis of both the severity of my problems and options that would be surgical and nonsurgical?
- Why have you made that prognosis and indicated those options?
- What will you do to determine the exact nature of my spinal problems?
- Do you have a team you generally work with on these types of surgeries?
- How many similar surgeries have you done, and what are the success statistics in detail?
- What do you recommend I do next?
- What do you see as a realistic scenario if I don't have surgery?
- Regarding exercise, at this point will pushing myself with physical activity be of any structural value or will it hurt me?
- Let each doctor know I will be getting other opinions and ask if there is someone he or she would recommend my seeing.
- If the doctor operates at a teaching hospital, ask who will actually be working on me.
- Ask for an initial reality check on timelines.
- Ask if I keep or get a copy of X-rays, tests, and so on I brought from the referring doctor as well as the ones you are having me get to take to other doctors.

I also wanted to let each doctor know a little about my health background. It seemed that might make a difference in how to proceed. I was completely open to either a male or female doctor, only concerned with locating the one who would do the most successful surgery, if I went ahead with such a drastic proposal. (At subsequent visits I became known as the lady with all the questions. I never ran out of them until much later.)

Soon I had a second opinion and some direction as to what to do next. Since more doctors followed, I'll refer to the original doctor I saw as Dr. Washington and his friend, who gave me the second opinion, as Dr. Adams.

Dr. Adams told me Dr. Washington may have been a bit dramatic, but there was no doubt that proceeding with the surgery would be the best way to stop the curvature from continuing and would minimize pain. He suggested that since Dr. Washington's X-rays were the first I'd had since my teenage years, they could be considered a baseline. If I had X-rays taken every six months, it would be easy to see how rapidly, or not, my spine and ribs were moving and torquing. He also pointed out that pain and disability would also indicate a negative change as well. "You need to get a CT and MRI so we can measure more accurately what is happening. You can make that appointment here and then come back to me and we'll go over the more detailed information." He thought, from the X-ray I had brought with me and his examination, I had a window of one to two years as the best timeframe, a balance between deterioration and my basic good health still intact. He said, as had Dr. Washington, "There is always a chance you will be able to keep some good quality of life without a surgery. The body is often very surprising." He encouraged me to stay as physically active as possible.

I made appointments for the CT scan and an MRI, which use different kinds of X-rays and equipment. The MRI didn't need special timing or dyes; I was just inside a noisy hollow tube, following directions to hold my breath, hold still, or relax. I don't get claustrophobic, but for people who do, the MRI can be difficult. If you don't have the extra money to go to a facility that has "open" MRI equipment, my suggestion to anyone with such concerns is to close your eyes when you are in the machine and use visualization to change your experience, which I did to make it better and more pleasant. I closed my eyes and visualized myself in warm tropical waters with flippers and a mask on, underwater and looking at coral and beautiful fish. The strange sounds from the machine were just muffled sounds from the boat and not important. Snorkeling or scuba diving is not something I have ever done, but because I have seen it on film, listened to people talk about it passionately, and read about it, I could imagine it easily. For me it turned the test into something more relaxing and also took my mind off the reason I was there.

A couple of weeks later I went back to Dr. Adams for the test results, which confirmed his original thoughts. He said, "You could make an appointment for the surgery now and do it next month. This would actually be two surgeries with a day of rest separating them." I know I must have looked stunned and probably horrified as well. I simply wasn't ready to deal with a surgery of such magnitude and wanted both more opinions and more options. Chiropractic massage and stretching exercises were still helpful and possible at that time, and I considered I might be one of those people who can keep on going regardless of what my spine might have started doing.

I found with both Dr. Washington and Dr. Adams that I was discussing "the spine" and "the situation" as though they were in a body other than mine. It seemed the easiest way to ask questions is to really listen and write everything down. But when I got out to my car or arrived home, the reality that this was really happening to me hit emotionally. It was tremendously difficult. I decided to turn the doctor trips into something more fun: go with a friend and pair the doctor visit with a happier activity.

By the end of my second week of the "new reality," I was feeling much better and stronger than I had the week earlier. It was still like being on a roller coaster, but at least for the time being I was on a level stretch. I thought, At least the second opinion isn't any worse than the first. I started to hear from friends about what they heard from friends of friends. Many were people with back problems and information they had found on the Internet. Perhaps, I thought, working my way through some of this would produce additional useful information for me.

It seemed strange that both doctors and many friends seemed surprised I had so many questions and that I was taking a very detailed approach to the situation. But to me it was the most obvious thing to do. *We were talking about my life. I don't know what else I have that is more valuable than that.* What would I be giving up to spend time coming to terms with this change in the direction of my life—watching television? Working overtime?

I went back to Dr. Washington, who gave me a cortisone shot. It released me from a lot of pain. I had started limping because of the subtle balancing act my body was going through. I knew the shot was not a long-term solution, but it bought me more time. Dr. Washington gave me names of two additional doctors who were out of state. He said, "Even the same X-rays will be read and interpreted differently by each doctor, and if you see enough doctors, you'll find the variety of answers doesn't end. You'll know when you have enough information to make your best decision. And if you don't, your spine and general health will make it for you." This is not a guy you'd want invite to a comedy club for laughs.

What lies behind us and what lies before us
are small matters compared to what lies within us.
—Ralph Waldo Emerson

CHAPTER 2

THE JOURNEY TOWARD SOLUTIONS

~⌒

A month later I was on my way north to see a doctor in Seattle. A friend took the day off work, and we planned to do some sightseeing before heading back from the day trip. I had an original X-ray with me and a CD with information on it. I had been told that doctors use their computers now for viewing rather than looking at cumbersome X-rays. But when I got to the doctor's office, he didn't have a computer and his nurse treated me like I had lost my mind when I handed her the CD. Very fortunate for me that my friend had her laptop and went into the doctor's office with me. Dr. Jefferson was almost more interested in the technology than with my dilemma. He had a sense of humor and said he did these surgeries when warranted, but there were other options. He suggested I continue to exercise, stay active, use the cortisone shots, and see how that worked. He said there were other types of less invasive surgeries to relieve pain I might want to consider at some point. "This extreme surgery should be the last resort" was his parting remark. I was glad to have someone else with me. Over lunch we discussed what I had heard and what she had heard, which made for more accurate notes. I was also able to express how it all made me feel, which was helpful, and wandering through Pike Place Market added a holiday feel to what might just have been an uneasy morning.

I had heard good things about a large medical center in California. A relative of a friend had seen a doctor there for another type of back issue and was really impressed with the facility's medical thoroughness. I got the doctor's name and phone number and called to make an appointment. I had already found out that each visit requires tons of paperwork and that even though it seems they all ask for the same information, I had to fill out the specific forms for each office. Keeping a copy of one form saved me a lot of time in completing the others. I told the appointment desk that I was coming from out of state and taking time off work to do so. I wanted to be sure the doctor would be there when I came to town. My hope was that if he was called into surgery, he would have a partner who would see me.

Two days before my appointment I got a call that the doctor would not be in the office and I would have to reschedule. Of course I had my airline reservation and a hotel booked. I was unhappy, not only because I had lost money on the hotel reservation and airline ticket but also because of the underlying tension involved in trying to get answers to questions I need answered but wish didn't even exist. I made the second appointment, again reiterating my out-of-state status. Three days before the appointment I got a cancellation call again. I was so angry that I had to wait a few days before I called back. I explained the problem and asked for suggestions regarding seeing someone who was well versed with my medical situation who would actually be able to see me when I was scheduled. I found out that trying to see a somewhat-famous doctor has its drawbacks.

The doctor I had been trying to see was booked on speaking engagements so often that the cancellations were not going to stop. I agreed that an almost-as-qualified doctor, who could actually see me, would meet my needs a lot better. By then I was booking my appointment for Thanksgiving weekend. It was a very happy turn of events for me that friends in the area invited me to stay for the weekend and also volunteered to drive to the appointment with me.

It not only helped defray costs—at least no hotel or rental car to deal with—but more important, gave me a safe and caring place to be while letting the doctor's recommendations settle in.

The fourth doctor, Dr. Madison, looked at a few of the X-rays and examined my spine. He nodded and responded, "The extreme surgery required to actually stop and correct your problems must be a last resort. In fact, you have two problems. The simpler one is disc deterioration, which is not so risky and would relieve much of the pain I expect you will soon be experiencing. But that surgery cannot be done without a huge negative impact to the rest of your back, which would also need to be corrected in a more hazardous surgery. I think exercise and the use of a custom-made brace would be your best bet for as long as possible." Again, having friends with whom I could talk this through, along with other pleasant activities and laughter, were critical to absorbing such frightening information and still go on with the everydayness of regular living.

Each doctor visit drilled into me the reality of how severe the problem really was. But I felt relieved to hear that there were lots of things I could still do that might lengthen the time between the now and a future surgery, maybe even eliminating the need for it. Doctors talked about the upcoming pain and disability, and although I heard what they were saying, I had too much denial of *coming to that* to apply it to an actual future that might be mine.

Taking a break from all the medical issues was my decision for the Christmas season. Traditionally, my family came home for the holidays and stayed at my house. We had a week of intense together-ness that long term could have gotten nasty, but in the short term was an intense coziness of emotion and activity. We talked only briefly about my information-gathering experiences, and they assured me they would be there for me however the scenario played out. All our intentions were genuine, and there was simply no way to really know what *being there for me* would require from anyone. In this secure set-ting, the possibility of surgery, disability, and life-changing physical and emotional issues all seemed very remote and unconnected to our special little family.

Toward the end of January I had another doctor appointment in Seattle. Dr. Washington assured me his recommendation to see Dr. Monroe would provide a great experience and would be able to explain the positive aspects of the surgery. When I checked with my friends to see if someone could drive up with me for the Friday appointment, I found a friend already with plans to spend that weekend in Seattle with her friend. I was invited to see an art exhibit of Frida Kahlo's paintings with a chance to shop and visit. I realized that even as the need for these medical evaluations had ominous overtones, they also created and allowed unexpected pockets of fun and adventure. We also discovered that a movie just released on the life of the artist was playing in Seattle as well. We planned to see the exhibit Saturday afternoon and the movie that evening.

Dr. Monroe checked my back and the X-rays. He appeared on the verge of tears and panic. He said, "This is a very hazardous surgery. Do you understand that nerves get cut and have to be reconnected? The spine is dismantled and put back together with material from your pelvic bone and marrow. This is a very lengthy surgery with a high complication rate. Yes, I have done these, but I won't do this surgery for you or anyone else again. Maybe my partner will. He has done pretty well with these. If at some point in the future you decide you really want to go through with this, let me know and perhaps my partner will see you to evaluate."

Abruptly, he left me in the examining room. I couldn't believe the conversation that had just taken place. I didn't even know how to start processing his comments because I had gone in with such a predetermined positive outcome in mind. How could there be such a disparity in these doctors' opinions?

The next day we enjoyed the beautiful Frida Kahlo paintings and were all looking forward to seeing the movie about this talented woman. We didn't know, at that time, that a large part of her life had been given over to serious back problems from a childhood accident and that she survived painful and not particularly helpful surgeries from that time on. The movie was riveting, and what she endured at the hands of doctors was horrific. I just sat in my seat as the credits rolled. Then, as we made our way up the aisle, my friend asked if I was OK and I said I was. But I wasn't. When we got to the lobby, the emotional weight of my situation really hit me completely. I stood facing the wall, sobbing uncontrollably. I couldn't stop crying and I couldn't let go of the wall. I don't know how long I stood there in that state. Thank goodness for friends who just let that be what I needed to do as they stood between me and the crowd leaving the theater.

The shuddering, uncontrollable crying was really cathartic. Not since my initial appointment with Dr. Washington had I dealt with my situation on an emotional level. I didn't realize the heaviness of that kind of denial until I was able to let it go. It was also a good lesson and a way to relook at what protecting myself really meant. Being vulnerable is sometimes the strongest thing to do.

When I returned home, I made an appointment with Dr. Washington and told him of my experience with Dr. Monroe. He responded, "I guess after lots of successes, he must have performed a surgery that really went badly." That was probably true but not very reassuring.

An X-ray was also taken at the six months mark to see if any major changes had taken place since the baseline X-ray. I learned that when reading an X-ray, there is much more to consider than what appears on the film. Posture, stance, and just the view of the reading physician can make a difference of several degrees when measuring degrees of change. My X-rays didn't indicate major changes but also couldn't tell us of minor ones. It seemed my best option would be to go on living my life and try some of the nonsurgical approaches suggested. The good news was that I had some time to do the things I wanted to do, including research, trying all kinds of relief, and viewing the need for surgery as a possibility in the future. I had the gift of time that someone who starts to cross the street and wakes up in the hospital with life changed forever doesn't have. I was grateful for that.

Six months after finding out the nature and direction of my physical pains and deformity, I was planning a trip to India, energetic in my job, and reading an amazing amount of material on the Internet about various sorts of spinal maladies and purported solutions. I was still exercising to videos at home, getting chiropractic massage, and, as they became gradually more difficult, paying attention to all the activities I had been taking for granted. Going to the park and spreading a blanket was an ideal way to read the Sunday paper. I enjoyed lying on my back watching clouds. Such an afternoon now also brought thoughts of how difficult it might be to get up off the blanket. By the end of that summer, I needed a hand to get up.

One of my lists contained those activities I wanted to be sure to do while I still could. Figuring that if my back stopped its downward spiral, the worst that could happen would be that I'd have even more time to do what I enjoyed. I'd have more time to experience what was important to me. I took my family to Las Vegas for Christmas, and we saw the Blue Man Group show, shopped, enjoyed the spas, and played together. The value of balance in being able to play, along with dealing with heavy issues, can't be minimized.

One of my long-time passions is traveling and particularly to faraway places, usually by myself. It is the combination of spontaneity, being a citizen not just of my own country but of the world, and feeling a sense of what a new place is about coupled with the sharing of it with others when I return that draws me. I planned the trip to India as realistically as I could, knowing I would need assistance and probably come up against physical limitations I didn't even know I had. The blessing of being adaptable meant quietly accommodating my home, work space, and activities to minimize my frailties. The downside was not realizing the degree of debilitation that had taken place. It is in the stretching outside the comfort zones where discovering reality takes place, if you want that.

Carol R. Palo

I went to India and was so glad for the experience. I had incredible opportunities to meet people, see a part of the world unknown to me, and bring back rich memories and growth as a person. I also came face-to-face with the degree of change in my physical condition. Even with a less arduous agenda than I would have undertaken in the past, I was surprised at how much pain I hadn't considered happening came from activities. Jeep rides over roads with potholes had me packing my back in ice each night to reduce the pain and swelling. Then came a time when nothing on this planet was worth seeing if it involved one more flight of stairs. Regardless of my desire or willfulness, at some point each day I had to stop and rest, no matter what it cut from the plans. Still, I had made the trip, was working as hard as ever, and enjoying the summer activities that were part of my interpretation of *summer with just a little extra help*.

The one-year mark from the first diagnosis arrived. The X-rays showed a drop of my rib cage towards my pelvis. The boyfriend disappeared, proving the adage that *difficulties aid a strong relationship and tear apart a weak one*. I started thinking about conserving my movements to avoid pain. The chiropractic massage and video workouts were becoming more pain provoking than helpful, and I started physical therapy. I also started reading up on my insurance, both health and long-term disability as well as company policy on taking a medical leave of absence. I still wasn't sure what I would be doing, but knowing what would be available to me was helpful. It was important for me to feel empowered, not victimized.

During my one-year checkup with Dr. Washington, we talked about the compression of bone into bone and what that would mean. I told him about my being able to travel but also about the pain I had started experiencing in my ribs, the regularity of difficulty both in getting up and walking.

He said, "These are classic symptoms. With more spinal torque and the drop of the rib cage, you'll experience more leg pain, more pressure on the nerves, and more rapid deterioration. How long do you want to wait? Do you still think you won't need surgery? How likely is that?"

I explained, "It's not that bad yet. I have financial considerations to deal with first. And, I'm not so convinced it will get that bad or that some other solution might not present itself as a permanent fix or at least to buy more time." Also, in all honesty, because I'd heard such a variety of thoughts from the doctors I'd seen, I wasn't sure what the best solution would be.

Dr. Washington responded, "OK, if you're not ready, a strong anti-inflammatory medication on a daily basis could help with any pains caused by the accompanying arthritis at least."

I went home and called a good friend and my family just to vent and get feedback. I went to bed thinking, I guess I'm OK. I just need to work, as a potential, on a presurgery to-do list and come up with a one- or two-year plan of what I'm going to do in case things really get as bad as Dr. Washington thinks. I went to sleep realizing it was Sept 10, the eve of the one-year anniversary of 9/11 and thought, There are bigger problems than mine.

The next six months could be called a short venture in physical therapy, the economics of enjoying but minimizing activities, planning another large trip, the fitting of the *I'll never wear that wretched thing* brace, and a very satisfying trip to California for the birth of my first grandchild. Oh, and I decided to buy a house.

Physical therapy was available because I had insurance that would cover it. Insurance is a wonderful thing. It makes possible treatments and medications that might otherwise be unaffordable. Finding doctors, facilities, and services that are covered in network or out of network, at 70% or 100% coverage, with and without annual or lifetime deductibles can be daunting. But I eventually found a physical therapist in my network. Her goal primarily was to see how active I could still be and then teach me exercises that would keep me as functional as possible for the longest period of time. We found I couldn't do much and usually left in so much pain that I could barely drive home.

It was very sobering to see how we had to keep scaling back what she wanted to teach me. She talked about exercises I needed to learn so I would be able get into a car. The process of sitting and swiveling to sit squarely in the seat was not something I had ever thought about, and the idea that it would soon be difficult was frightening.

Based on the suggestion from Dr. Madison, Dr. Washington sent me to have a custom- fitted brace. Even after two fittings it was hard to imagine what the final brace would look like. I returned to pick it up not knowing what to expect, but it certainly wasn't the hard-shell plastic and Velcro getup that my current wardrobe wouldn't fit over.

"I'll never wear this!" I howled out of sheer terror, not thinking of the hard work and pride the brace-maker and taken producing it.

"Yes you will when you hurt bad enough!" he snarled.

I took the brace home and put it in the back of a closet. I worked extra hard on my exercises.

Just before Christmas I got the call from my daughter saying that her water just broke. I was so grateful that I could still physically pack a bag, get on the airplane, and be present for the birth. I was also able to stay for weeks to help with this new wonderful baby girl. As I walked up and down their stairs with her, I noted how fortunate it was that this little girl was only six pounds. By then, lifting anything with real weight was very difficult. I was able to really enjoy the experience and be of help with housework, but it was arduous in a way I knew it wouldn't have been even a year earlier.

When I came home it seemed natural to start assessing my everyday living with the question, *if the pain gets lots worse and if I need surgery, how will I do this?* My little condo was easy to clean but small enough so I used all the space from floor to ceiling. How would I reach what I needed? The idea of an attached garage became very appealing, since I couldn't carry heavy bags of groceries anymore and so was making several trips up and down multi-stairways.

I found myself driving around on weekends looking at houses until I found just the right situation. For me that was a large, light, airy house with minimal yardwork, one well-padded flight of stairs, an attached double garage on property I felt sure would appreciate and give me a little more financial security. It was also wonderfully distracting to start such a positive venture and have the opportunity to pick out paint, carpet, and various finishes and watch something be built versus my own deterioration.

I thought I could handle one more adventuresome trip. Brazil, with its famous beaches, the Amazon jungle, and giant waterfalls along the Argentina border seemed like a grand way to say *maybe this will need to be the last big trip, and that's all right.*

The physical therapy, even at the minimal level we had set, was so painfully distracting that I gave it up. I focused instead on video workouts I could still modify to fit my ability. I walked a lot. Planning to sell my condo, I also attempted to sort out, clean, and prepare for a move. It's amazing what can be amassed in fourteen years. The trips up and down the stairs with the heavier items became too painful, and I started to ask friends to assist. I also let my family know that on their next visits they'd be put to work.

One and one-half years after finding out about my back condition, ground was broken on my new house and I had about thirty days to get ready for my trip to Brazil. I figured that when I returned I'd have to get serious about moving and find out what would be needed to sell my condo.

Brazil was everything I'd hoped for. I wandered the beaches in Rio and stood in the roaring spray of the amazing waterfalls of Igauzu. I received some seriously needed lessons on asking for help in the Amazon. I was reminded I could choose to enjoy the pleasures that came even when they were not from the choices I would have made. It was an arduous journey to get to the rustic resort in the Amazon basin, and activities were scheduled from early morning to late at night. I didn't want to pass up anything or ask for help even though I was exhausted and hurting. It was predictable that I would take a tumble, since pain and exhaustion now brought balance issues. My ego was more injured than my body, although a large, impressive bruise appeared later and I found out there were Anaconda in the river I had fallen into. People had offered to give me a hand into the boats, up the stairs, and so on, but until then I was too prideful. I learned to be more gracious about accepting a hand and even asking for it if needed. I had to pass on several activities and determine that if I wanted to enjoy the trip I would have to focus on what I could do, not bemoan what I could no longer do. These were two skills that became incredibly useful as my condition worsened.

When I returned home, a friend suggested I try to sell my condo myself. It was fortunate that the ad I placed brought someone who would buy the condo as is—I didn't even have to clean it and still received a fair price, which left me free to focus on my new home and the move.

Two years after originally hearing about the perils of my spinal condition, I moved into my new house and was ready to have an open house to celebrate. It was memorable, partly because it was fun to share a happy occasion with friends but also because it marked the beginning of a new phase of back debilitation. Everything was ready for my guests. As I was changing into nicer clothing, I developed incredible pain that felt like extreme pressure on a nerve. Ice had become my best friend in relieving and numbing pains, but there wasn't time. I had almost thrown out the dreaded brace when I moved, but I remembered where I had tossed it. I put it on under my clothing, and it provided enough relief to navigate the stairs and make it through the afternoon. The brace was becoming my new best friend.

That fall it became clear Dr. Washington's predictions were coming true. I fell at work and was not able to move until ice had numbed my back and I had taken more over-the-counter pain medication than should be taken. At home I attempted to lift my leg to walk up the stairs but I fell and had to be taken to the emergency room. It was pretty terrifying when an emergency room doctor looked at my back and stammered, "My God! I've never seen anything like this before!" As the ice stopped working, the brace and the drugs in as small doses as possible became the only solution.

I now found myself physically uncomfortable in so many situations that had been part of my life that I was gradually withdrawing from an active social life, which got a little quieter and my world a little smaller. However, I was still not ready to seriously commit to a risky surgery. I considered *bending like the willow*. Maybe there was some unseen value in letting my body have its way and letting my life be whatever would come from that, or maybe the surgery would be very successful, leading me to a fuller life. But what I was really waiting for was *the third choice*. Even though intellectually I knew there was none, at some deeper level I had not accepted that reality.

Close friends in Palm Springs invited me to spend a long weekend with them. I hadn't traveled since spring, and nine months later wasn't sure how I would handle a trip. But I wanted to give it a try. A friend took me to the airport. No parking in the economy lot and taking the shuttle to the airport this time. I had arranged for a wheelchair to take me from check-in onto the plane, and I needed it. I couldn't have walked all the way to the gate or even lift my travel bag for the security scanners. I chose an airline that had a direct flight and that was less than three hours long. A wheelchair escort and my friends were waiting at the other end, and so I could still travel. But I hadn't realized how little tolerance I really had left physically. My friends had tile floors in their home and my body was used to thick carpet. Standing and walking were painful. The bed was too hard for my tender body, and I couldn't sleep. I spent half the time on pain medication lying on a guest bed with comforters and pillows under me. I was still glad to see my friends, however. We visited and did some sightseeing, but it was quite a wake-up call regarding how much my body had changed in a year.

I found that being honest with technicians and doctors really created better situations for me. Dr. Adams accepted that I would often be in his office, each time with a new list of questions. He answered them all respectfully. In the process I developed trust in him and his ethics, a sense of knowing him as a person, and respect for his skills. He was able to see me as a complete person beyond the spinal X-rays. That knowledge, I think, allowed him to make surgical decisions later that gave me the best results for the life I hoped to be living.

When I was having a new procedure, I would let the nurses or technicians know if I was nervous or had questions. Having person-to-person dialogue was a better choice than whining or just being angry with fear and the impersonal nature of testing. I believe the experiences went more smoothly than they might have. It's not uncommon to be treated like one more *thing to do* in the course of the day when you are part of the stream of people being tested or treated. In early March I had an MRI. In one situation, as I lay on the table getting set up for the dye, a technician called others over saying, "Look at this back; have you ever seen anything like this?" I reminded them, "I'm here, too" and got an apology and perhaps a little extra TLC.

The turning point came, the moment when I knew in my gut there were only two choices—and really only one—I could make. It came in Dr. Adams's office when he and the technicians showed me the results of the MRI. As we viewed each slide, they explained what I was seeing. First was the symmetric circle of cord and nerves at the upper parts of my back. As the view moved down to the middle thoracic area, the symmetry became a piece of abstract art. I could see the curves and the clumping compression of nerves; everything looking much like a bad cubist painting. I felt a tremendous amount of compassion for my poor body. It was obvious how hard my muscles were working to keep me upright, clear why there was so much pain and disability when I looked at nerves in all the wrong places. No wonder technicians and doctors were aghast at what my body looked like. One of the medical residents who reviewed the slides with me gently pointed out there was no doubt where it was all headed. I knew then that the kindest thing I could do for me and for anyone who cared about me was to have the surgery.

Still, I wanted to talk to one of the other doctors I had initially contacted. My situation had clearly worsened, and I was hoping either for confirmation that I was making the best decision or that he might offer my last hope for a third choice. I had been impressed with Dr. Jefferson and so made an appointment. But his viewpoint shifted dramatically. He said, "I'm not so sure the large increase in pain is really from the scoliosis, and I don't know if the surgery will relieve that pain and pressure." He recommended another direction that included tests and injections. He gave me a brochure on the subject and asked me to let him know if that was the direction I wanted to go in. I was initially stunned and excited. It sounded as though the third option had just materialized!

I read the material and felt less elated. Bone scans, radiation, and in-hospital treatments of injections costing thousands of dollars each time was the course of action suggested. Even if the pain was relieved, it sounded like a Band-Aid approach, not a course of action that could be an actual solution. As I was leaving Dr. Jefferson asked, "You're here because you want to get rid of the pain, aren't you?" I realized that, of course I wanted freedom from the pain, but more than that, I wanted a real solution. I knew then that I was willing to accept the surgical risk as my solution.

Carol R. Palo

The purpose of life is to live it, to taste experience to the utmost, to reach out eagerly and without fear for newer and richer experience.
—Eleanor Roosevelt

CHAPTER 3

COMING TO TERMS WITH SURGERY: THE PROCESS

᠆᠆᠆᠑

*D*uring my next visit with Dr. Adams, I asked if I could talk to patients who had been through a similar surgery, preferably women around my age. He gave me the phone numbers of two patients who agreed to talk with other potential surgical candidates. I called the patients; they were incredibly honest and willing to answer all my questions. It was very reassuring to hear their stories and realities of going through the surgery and recovery process.

Now it was a matter of setting up a surgery date. I was torn between the desire to just get it done versus putting it off as long as I could. However, neither would have been a good decision.

On New Year's Day I had taken some time to go through all the notes I'd taken during doctor visits. Then I went through them again along with the acupuncture, physical therapy, and travel notes on all that was going on in my ever-diminishing world. It was clear that Dr. Washington's comments were true. The predictions of ribs pushing into the pelvis, extreme pain, and disability in probably two years had materialized. Next would come the inability to get to work regularly, disability, and a wheelchair. Then life would continue to get harder. Surgery was necessary and probably couldn't wait much more than seven or eight months, so I needed to find just the right time. The prime consideration would be when the surgeon and his team had time in their schedule. Next I needed to know when my family would be available for the longest period of time. Then I looked at my job responsibilities. I wanted to plan a smooth transition while I was gone, assuming I would be returning to work. It would also need to be a time in the annual work cycle that would be least busy. At the end of the list I visualized the weather—getting to the hospital, people being able to visit me, summer vacations or winter storms creating problems. If I could get on the doctor's schedule early, I would have some choices in surgery dates. My son was a teacher so July or August were good months for him. At work, February through June were the busiest times. When I called my surgeon's scheduler, I told myself quietly, I can always cancel, but I made a commitment to have the surgeries in mid-August.

At four months before surgery, it seemed my to-do list and questions just kept increasing.

I needed to put my affairs in order. I didn't have a will or even a health care directive. In the past it seemed that if I didn't have them then nothing would happen to me. That was foolish, of course, and now dangerous. I contacted an attorney and started the paperwork. At work I quietly started a one-year plan to roll out projects and expenditures. I considered who would take over each project or activity and who would cover my other responsibilities. I knew I couldn't predict the unpredictable, but I could put in motion a schedule that avoided chaos. I started conversations with my family about the surgery date and what would follow. I listened to them, just as important as giving them information and maybe more so, because they had lots of questions and concerns.

Whatever our beliefs are about an afterlife, God, the cosmos, and more, we all logically know we won't be on this planet as people forever. Our loved ones won't, either. Still, it's emotionally difficult to look at a parent you have viewed as strong, resilient, likely to be going strong for many, many more years and realize how fragile that all can be. I really didn't want to put my children in that position, but that was the reality and it would have been disrespectful, dishonest, and unkind to withhold information and not ask for their assistance.

My son lived out of state and visited every few months. My daughter, her husband, and their baby had moved back to town a year earlier. They knew, more than I realized, how the deformities in my back were changing how I lived and the level of pain I was in. Still, as we talked about my decision to have the surgery and all it involved, there was a sense of the unthinkable about to happen. They had questions. Was there a chance I could die? Might I be mentally damaged after the surgery? Might I be a vegetable? If the surgery went well, would I be normal again? What kind of help would I need immediately after surgery and for how long? Would I be able to work again? How long and in what way would I need assistance from them, specifically? They requested more details about the surgery. They needed reassurance regarding how I came to the decision.

Then there was the question of what to say or do about my mother. She was now in her mid-nineties and suffering from dementia. At Thanksgiving dinner at my house the prior fall, she had not recognized a photo of her and my dad that was taken when they were in their late fifties. After returning to her apartment in assisted living, she bemoaned to the staff that no one had come to see her for the holiday, forgetting that only hours before she had been having dinner with us. Those moments would come and go. She knew us all and was often able to keep track of when I came to visit her. She often told me she would be lost without my help and the time we spent together. I knew I wouldn't be able to visit for a long time even if the surgery went very well, and what if it didn't? We made a videotape to play for mom in case I didn't make it or was left in a state of being unable to visit her. The tape was just a warm, brief message stating that I loved her and was sorry I couldn't be visiting her. We agreed that if she asked, my son and daughter would say I was unable to come by, and when I was able to talk on the phone I would call and say I missed her and loved her but was working overtime, or had a bad cold—anything to avoid needlessly causing her stress and worry.

The questions my children raised were addressed during the next visits I had with Dr. Adams. My daughter started joining me on those visits, which was really helpful. Having friends to debrief with had been so much better than dealing with the whole process on my own. Now, with a surgery date set, there was no longer a boundary line between discussing the spine and attaching the process to me as a person. Having her with me was both emotionally soothing and practical in setting a plan of action.

This list of questions for the doctor came next:

- Would I be able to use stairs, and how long after a successful surgery would that be? (My bedroom was upstairs.)
- Would I be able to do basic skills like put on my socks, wipe myself in the bathroom, take a shower by myself, move my arms overhead, and dress myself?
- Having been told I would be put in a brace right after surgery, what kind of brace would it be and how long would I be in it?
- Since I lived alone, would I be self-sufficient enough to go home directly from the hospital?
- If family or a friend were able to come by every day, would that be enough help?
- What therapies would I need to become as functional as possible?

As I tried to think ahead, I felt I would never run out of questions. It was not so much trying to stay in control of events I would have little control over, but it was wanting to set up a scenario that would be manageable for those taking care of me. It was a way to make sure the financial concerns such as insurance needs were taken care of, too. I also wanted to do all I could to ensure I would have a job to come back to.

I knew surgery precertification and lots of forms to complete would be required. I wanted some idea of how much I would need to pay after insurance covered its portion. I had signed up for long-term disability insurance when I first started my job. It cost only a few dollars each month. How much would it pay and what information did it need to start the process? From the doctor's comments, I knew it would be best for me to go to a rehabilitation center for a while after surgery. I would need someone to help me turn from side to side every two hours and at some point help me get steady on my feet to make it to the bathroom. I would make long-term gains if occupational therapy were available every day. Having professional assistance in regaining balance walking and adding strength would help me become self-sufficient sooner.

After contacting an attorney and having a will drawn up, I obtained the state's advance directives form used in case a patient is unable to speak. It asks for the name of your spiritual advisor, your doctor, what medical treatment you want or don't want regarding life support, who can speak for you, and other questions that no one really wants to discuss with loved ones. I found the conversation and completion of the paperwork very difficult for my family and me. But it also brought us peace of mind. If that undesired scenario were to happen, there would be no angst in guessing what should or shouldn't be done.

By May I was wearing the brace under my clothing all the time except at night. Most of my energy was spent just trying to do my job and the basics of living. It became common for me to rush home from work, eat quickly, take pain medication, and hurry to my bedroom before the pain and inability to lift my legs became so great that I couldn't make it up the stairs. It was clear that scheduling the surgery was a good choice. The question was more a matter of how to stay functional until mid-August. I also needed to let my boss and close coworkers know what was coming. I knew they would want me to have a plan regarding how my duties would be divided and what projects would be worked on, especially if I planned on returning to work.

I met with my boss and told him I had been experiencing serious back problems and would need surgery. It was set for August, and I had a plan to have all duties and projects covered. He was stunned when I told him I wouldn't be back for probably seven months, but could probably work part time from home after three or four months. I held my breath to hear what he would say. Seven months is a long time. I hadn't even said that that scenario would be under the best of outcomes. He asked me to present a plan with some specifics he added, and I knew then there was at least a good chance my job would not be given to someone else permanently. It is fortunate there are current job protection laws, but they generally are effective for twelve weeks. Not everyone is as fortunate as I was in such a situation.

The person who would be overseeing my duties, my boss, and I worked out a plan of how my job would be divided. Because I had talked to my doctor about what I might realistically do under the most successful of outcomes, I was able to present a tentative schedule of when I would be able to work from home a few hours a day and what type of work I would be able to do. We planned for a phased-in return to duties, gradually adding hours and specific tasks and projects until I could start to work in the office. We also phased in returning to the workplace, adding hours and days until I would be in the office full time. Psychologically, this plan was very reassuring not only to me but to my employer and coworkers, who could see a process and completion of necessary work.

My conversations with the doctor and two of his satisfied patients, and information on the Internet made clear that life was not going to revert to the way it had been, even under the best circumstances. Stretching, bending, and twisting my back would be minimal. Bending would be at the hips only. Two days of surgery stress on my body and brain carried risks. Cutting so many nerves and trying to reattach them all might not be successful, which could easily leave me with some paralysis or limited vision. Rebuilding the spine and hoping it would all fuse properly would require the surgeon's best skills and the patient's absolute resolution and cooperation. The question for me was, *How do I make peace with whatever the surgery brings?*

As I was able to check off the practical questions and tasks, I found myself in need of emotional and spiritual direction as well. I had been aware of the benefits of finding strength, freedom from stress, calmness, and acceptance from such things as meditation, being out in nature, and visualizing. I had tried all of them, often with gratifying results, but never as though my life truly depended on them. As I talked to people who had been through difficult times, I realized that my life, at least the quality of it, would be shaped by my ability to practice meditation and visualization. I read books, talked to people, and tentatively tried to open my mind to what I would need to do at a practical level. It came down to some simple actions: three basic choices and all worked for me, just providing different sorts of good results.

1. I stepped out of doors to enjoy nature. I walked or stood for a while, or sometimes just sat. All I had to do was focus on nature, really seeing each leaf or cloud, smelling the damp in the air or the pine needles, feeling the breeze and the sun on my skin. This kind of meditation refreshed and relaxed me and helped me to feel part of a large, good something.

2. I sat or lay down and focused on breathing slowly and regularly. When thoughts or emotions entered, I noted only that they were there but refocused more on the breathing as though unhurried, even breathing were the only thing in the world I needed to do. The result was usually release from physical and mental tension.

3. I visualized in great detail an ideal location. I could even feel the sand between my toes and hear the ocean at a distance, like taking a mini vacation.

Although the visualization seemed more like a little treat than serious meditation, it turned out to be the vehicle that guided me to the inner and outer peace I would need to go into surgery and beyond.

My Life as a Metal Sculpture

I started looking for easy opportunities to take these mini vacations, usually occurring Saturday and Sunday mornings on my patio in the Oregon summer sun. It was easy to relax and visualize myself on a beach blanket, warm sand crunching around my heels, and the ocean's soft roar rolling over me. In thinking of the ocean, I was reminded of the cosmic ocean meditation I had read about—being a little wave among many waves all on, in, and a part of the ocean. I found, over the weeks, that the sense of being a part of the water or even being on water was directing my visualization. It was changing into less of me imagining what was coming next and more of me going along for the ride.

We all have the capacity to find our own meditation-visualization vehicle to travel through a rough and strange time. The following is what came to me and worked for me presurgery, the earliest recovery days, and during the long rehabilitative period:

> I am on a river. It is so quiet I can hear the
> reeds almost parting as the boat slides into the
> water. It is so quiet that if there were a gnat or a fly
> I could hear its wings move, but there is no insect.
> The air seems to have its own weight. I am on a
> small, sparse boat. I sit on the wooden seat in the
> back, with my hands in my lap. There is no need
> or desire to do anything except sit and note that
> my guide, in a hooded cloak with his back to me,
> is using a pole to move us into the river. There is
> no one else in the boat. I know this is not a round
> trip. I will not come back to whom or where I was
> before. We may land very close to that spot or far
> away. There is no way to know. There will be people
> I know along the way. I will not see them. They
> are not at the river's edge, but they are there for
> me. Wherever we land is where I will go on with
> my life, whatever it turns out to be. There is no

Carol R. Palo

cause for concern. It will just be who and where I
am. There is no need to feel anything. All that is
required of me is to be.

I returned to my backyard patio after each of these visualization-
meditation experiences feeling more relaxed, calmer, and more connected to everything.

By my birthday in July, the countdown of days until surgery had
begun. It's interesting that after I determined I was going to have the
surgery, I didn't want to know anymore facts about it. I think I had
divided up who does what: The surgery's success was my doctor's
business. Advocating for me, during the times when I couldn't, was
picked up by my son and daughter. My role was to be a good patient.

Back to the checklists of what still needed to be done.

By four weeks prior to surgery, there was no more room for thinking it was somewhere in the future. I made sure my will, temporary
power of attorney, and medical instruction forms were completed
and that my children knew where they were.

Then came the last doctor's appointment. My daughter attended
with me so we could both ask our questions. What is the check-in
procedure? What should I bring? Neither of us asked what to do if
everything goes wrong. We had family talks on the phone since my
son needed to know when to come and for how long to stay initially.
Names and phone numbers of my close friends were available to help
my children as well as me through the ordeal. I double-checked with
the insurance company and had a list of rehab centers that would be
covered by my insurance.

I know there were many phone calls between my son and daughter
I never knew about, and my son-in-law geared up to have no spare
time since he would draw the job of babysitting duty and morale
support. My close friends were so supportive, and I knew they would
be in the hospital room with me to hold my hand, pray for recovery,
and hug my children. I stayed on at work until just a few days before
surgery. There seemed to be so much to get done and transfer over.

It was also good to have something to focus on besides the surgery and what would come next.

A few years earlier I had seen Mom go through terrorizing hallucinations on morphine after her hip replacement surgery. It scared me. I also talked to people who had morphine after surgery and read up on it a little—being under anesthetic for an extended time can cause mental damage as we get older, and that scared me, too. I was assured by my doctor that I could express my concerns directly to the anesthesiologist, who would be very careful to put me under to just the right degree. I also asked that morphine be used only for as long as it was absolutely necessary. I wanted assurance that I wouldn't have the same terror as my mom had to take with me into surgery and that strange period right after. I needed a sense that I would be calm and okay whatever strangeness might be waiting for me.

Three days before surgery I wrote the following:

> The gift of a deteriorating physical condition,
> which for me is the combination of moving sco-
> liosis with arthritis, also contains an extraordinary
> adventure. I find I am in the midst of it, much
> like trips I have taken to Greenland, Morocco, and
> China. There is a sense of need and desire to go to
> this place and the checking out of data—cost, time,
> possibilities, gains, losses. Can I? Will I?

Then comes the setting in motion—the factual actions, the schedule, payments, time allotments in place, what do I need for the travels, what needs to be done beforehand at home, what will be waiting for me when I return. Each trip has a great sense of adventure and happiness. Each trip has a point in time when I ask myself, "What in blazes are you doing? It's expensive, you're all alone, it's all unknown, blah blah blah blah." I turn it off and it fades away to be replaced by the adrenalin of readiness.

The entire trip process—from initial sense of "I could go there" 'til I pull up in my driveway afterward—changes who I am and who

Carol R. Palo

I return as. Each adventure has special bonuses that come from it. This adventure is no different. I am only partway through, but have already received:

- Healthy body image. Like most girls and women in our society, the critical body-image eye develops early, and there are few who are comfortable with the way their bodies look and feel. I was no exception. But after I saw the MRI and my twisted spine—nerves jammed into odd-shaped spaces and bones pushing into bones—I developed a real compassion and respect for my body. I really looked at it differently, too. I am proud of it and can see not only the deformities but also the grace, curves, softness, and strength of those poor muscles that work so hard to keep me upright and minimize the pain. This body that houses me deserves a chance to be straightened and function as best as is possible.

- The grace of less self-reliance. Out of necessity has come the ability to ask for help (at least some improvement), and with that has come a real letting go and an allowing of people to assist—and in their own way. A good example is my little garden. If I had the money and physical ability, I would have paid for, designed, and taken care of a nice little garden. But I didn't have a lot of money, little plant knowledge, and no ability to do any planting or plant care. A series of visits from friends, each whom I thanked as I could by offering coffee, cooked a meal, paid for expenses, or just said, "Thank you, this means so much to me," resulted in a wonderful and surprising result. The collaboration of my ideas plus their ideas, elbow grease, plant-garden knowledge, and generosity resulted in a beautiful garden, which is better than anything I could have put together on my own. The bonus is that whenever I am on the patio I not only enjoy the garden but also think of all the beautiful people who put it together.

- Slowing down. Pain is a great redirector of attention. It moved me toward the value of purposeful breathing, the art of just

My Life as a Metal Sculpture   37

breathing and being, the being in each moment, and feeling all the dimensions of it.

- Values. I looked again at where I spend my energy. Dealing with pain requires lots of energy. Energy spent on self-pity, anger, or fear is wasted energy. Energy is better spent reclaiming love, laughter, and cosmic consciousness.
- The beautiful umbrella of family and friends. I was able to let go and know they've got my back and everything else that matters.

The surgery was scheduled for a Monday morning, and I didn't have to check in the night before. First I thought it would be one last night to go with friends or family, but I spent most of the night in the bathroom. I hadn't considered that I would be taking diuretics to completely clean out my system. No food, beverages, just cleaning out my system. It was still cleaning out on the way to the hospital. Whatever false sense of bravado I might have planned on displaying, soiling myself while checking into the hospital was a pretty sure sign that my body was no longer my own but part of the process I was about to participate in.

While I was in bed and waiting for the anesthesiologist, my son and daughter waited with me, filling the time with small talk and joking, which seemed to be the best thing to do at such a strange time. Then the doctors appeared and we talked about anesthesia, not too much but certainly not too little, either. Cutting me open from the front, moving some organs, and doing prep work—the shorter five-hour surgery—would happen that morning. The next day they would see how my body handled the anesthetic. The second, longer surgery on my back would be done on Wednesday, taking six to ten hours depending on *how it goes*. I was told I would be heavily sedated for Tuesday, the interim twilight day. They gave me a shot to relax me, and while I waited for them to finish wheeling me down the hall, I was out. I had wondered what it would be like to lay in the operating room waiting for the anesthetic to take effect; that's what I had seen in movies. Mercifully, for both surgeries I was out before we even got close to the operating room.

～◯

Coming to, slowly, was more a sense than actually seeing or hearing. I was aware my son, daughter, and a few close friends were in the room. It was evident the first surgery had been completed since I was alive and thinking, and not feeling too bad but aware my body had just been through something massive. I knew I was full of morphine. The room was full of ghostlike people I called the shadow people. They didn't seem to be bothering me, and I was able to remind myself that they were only a product of the morphine so there was nothing to fear about them, anyway. At some point I heard people speaking and I sometimes bothered to respond, but I don't know if any actual sounds or words came out. It seemed to me I was asked how I felt, and friends made sure I could see they were there. Did we converse in anyone's actuality except mine? I don't know. It doesn't matter.

It was clear to the doctors, to my family and friends, and even to me that I had done pretty well and that there would be the larger, second one on Wednesday. I recall being in another conversation about the anesthetic and another trip down the hall to the operating room. When I next realized I was back in my room, I knew both surgeries were done.

I had been face down for the longer, second surgery, and apparently blood had pooled and my body had bloated—a standard reaction, as we were told later. I remember, sometime during the first three or four days, seeing the plastic identification bracelet on my wrist. When I checked into the hospital and it was put on, it almost slid off my small wrist. Now it was almost imbedded in my skin and wasn't going anywhere. Later I found out that when my children had been paged that I was on my way back from surgery, they saw a bed containing a very fat, bloated body full of tubes being brought to my room. They pointed out that a patient was being delivered to the wrong room, that it was their mother's room. The nurses checked the wrist bracelet and said, "This is her." I can't imagine how horrific it must have been for them not to even recognize their own mother. I had the easy role of just lying in bed, realizing that for some reason there was a lot more of me.

As the anesthesia wore off, I became more able to sort through the morphine fog and assess what was going on. Beautiful floral arrangements had arrived and were still arriving. The flowers were important to me. They were something beautiful to focus on and reminded me that I was cared about. It seems to me either my son or daughter or both were by my bed most of the days. I remember food being brought and being helped to eat, although I don't recall having any appetite or even if the food was tasty. I am normally known as a lover of quality chocolate and little boxes of chocolate also appeared. It was shocking to discover that the very sight and scent of chocolate made me nauseated. I think that startled my friends almost as much as my physical appearance did.

I received lots of unanticipated gifts during the journey of surgery and rehabilitation. One came just a few days after surgery while I was still in the hospital. It was evening or night and I had been dozing when I became aware that someone was by my bedside, talking to me. The person, perhaps thinking I was asleep or unconscious, poured his heart out to me, with dreams, hopes and fears, and asked for direction. My first thought was, What are you doing! I've just had surgery and I can't help anyone. I can't even move. But then I realized I could be of help. I just listened and allowed this person to say things out loud he needed to say. It surprised me to realize that even though I was almost physically helpless, it didn't make me any less valuable or useful. The gift of empowerment in such a condition was pretty amazing.

Over the next few days I became more aware of my surroundings, the nurses, visitors, and excruciating trips to X-ray. I started recalling the enormity of the surgeries and how many nerves had been cut and reconnected. I was told there would be some temporary or even permanent residuals. My right hand felt quite numb. The grace of the drug haze allowed me to be only concerned, not panicked; my drugged mind assessed that I was right handed, but it was probably temporary and I had another hand anyhow.

As the time to leave the hospital grew closer, the staff insisted that I sit up at the edge of my bed to transfer to a chair and take a few steps. Now I discovered that my left leg had forgotten how to take commands from my brain. It just didn't do anything when I wanted it to move. The physical therapist gave me directions to reactivate the pathways between the brain and leg. It was really interesting to teach my leg to obey, sort of as though it had become an obstinate pet. I was coached to slap my leg and say "Move" out loud if it helped. When that didn't work, I was told to yell at it and cuss if necessary, whatever it took to get my leg's attention. I could feel the connection being remade, much more quickly than I thought would happen. It was less than ten days, I think, before I could think Move! strongly and the leg cooperated. I had never thought about those body movements prior to my back problems; I had taken them for granted. I was very humbled with my little inconvenience when I thought of those with spinal cord injuries and paralysis who couldn't yell and slap their limbs back into motion.

My experience in the hospital allowed me to note that the staff all had the same goal I had, and that was to get me out of the hospital as soon as was reasonable. The difference was everyone's definition of *reasonable*. It seemed to me the doctors looked primarily at how their incisions were healing and how to best keep any infections from setting in. For those reasons they wanted me out quickly. The nurses had a checklist and needed it completed prior to checkout. That is the only reason I can think of for them to ask someone heavily medicated, "Have you had a bowel movement in the last two days?" I had no idea, and when prompted, "Do you think you might have?" the answer "Maybe" got a swift check mark and a "Good for you. You know you can't leave until you've had a BM." The physical therapists needed me to sit, move a couple of steps, and reseat myself before they could say their job was completed. The first therapist, I think, must have gotten his training in the military. He barked orders at me. He challenged, he stared, he pushed. It was probably a great technique for some patients, but not for me. After a couple of sessions, my heart started palpitating and I needed to be put on oxygen. He just scared me, and I felt too pressured to even think about actually moving. The second therapist was more of a coach and encouraged me. This approach was better for me, and I was able to accomplish the transfer to a chair, although it was very scary and painful.

No one appeared to be considering the reasonableness of where I would go. Who would take care of me? Was I really physically and emotionally ready for the transition? Was I being pushed too hard or not enough? This is when the importance of having someone to advocate comes in.

Because I had talked to my doctor and insurance company at length prior to surgery, I knew I would need to go to a rehabilitation center before going home. I needed more care than my son and daughter were able to provide, including daily occupational and physical therapy that would speed my recovery and aid my spirit. I had a list of facilities in my area that insurance would pay for. As soon as both surgeries were completed, and some rough idea of how long I might be in the hospital was available, my son checked nursing homes online, then picked the two with the highest ratings. He went to both facilities unannounced and just sat in the lobby, observing the interaction among the staff, patients, and visitors. At one there was no interaction. No one was smiling, and patients sat unattended and expressionless in the hallway. At the other staff and patients were chatting with one another, and staff asked my son what he needed. Arrangements were made for me to stay at the more pleasant of the two, which was also the only one to offer some type of therapy seven days a week. In addition, the location was ideal. It was close to my daughter's house and close to where many of my friends lived. My daughter would be the one to see me daily since my son had to go back to work for a while. My daughter was a mom working full-time, so having me close made it easier for her. It also gave me great peace of mind to know how close she was. Being in a nursing home for three to five weeks seemed like it would be more bearable with visitors, and the location made that more likely. The problems were making arrangements, getting the final insurance approval, and making sure of bed availability, which could take a few days. I was in no position to advocate for myself, so my son did. He met with both doctors and administrators, but he had to fight hard to get me two extra days in the hospital. No one disagreed that I was immobile, very fragile, and needed to have an appropriate place to go, but the checklists had all been completed so to them that meant I should leave. Dr. Adams had been called out of town; he might have been able to write an order for the delay. I am also very grateful I had those extra days because just being moved, even by ambulance, was very painful, exhausting, and traumatic.

Of course I wanted to leave the hospital. It was a good sign that I was truly in the process of reclaiming my life. The rehab center would offer a little more independence and would teach me the skills I needed for the next phase, which was going home. But I was also afraid to leave the hospital, which had skilled people who knew me and were constantly there to actively take care of me, people who knew what my difficulties were. Of course my body was very fragile. I had to be turned from one side to the other every two hours, and pillows kept at my back. I could not sit up or try to get up without a special brace. It seemed complex to get into and came with an instruction sheet that I wasn't sure anyone would really read. My left leg was just starting to work, the lower part still swollen. The three middle toes of my right foot didn't seem to want to hold my weight well, and my right hand was numb. And then there was my voice—more a matter of not having a voice. I was told the intubation tube had scratched my larynx, not uncommon, and the voice almost always returned. I could say a few words at an almost normal sound level, and it would rise or fall without my having any control until the sound disappeared entirely. Sometimes I would open my mouth and no sound came out at all. I felt so helpless; worst of all, it seemed to me, was the inability to call for help.

I left the hospital with a parade of flowers, a nicely framed family photo, and a small gift box of chocolates (the smell still nauseated me, but I believed the day would come when I would be eating chocolates again with gusto). I think my daughter rode in the ambulance with me and my son waited at the nursing home. Even though I had been given extra drugs for the ride and the attendant said he was driving quite slowly and carefully, it was an exhausting trip; I was relieved just to be placed in a bed I could call my own.

At first dreams seem impossible, then improbable, then inevitable.
—Christopher Reeve

CHAPTER 4

THE REHABILITATION CENTER

~)

I was in a semiprivate room. The woman in the bed next to me was about fifteen years older than I and rehabilitating from foot problems. She had been in the facility another time and, apparently had been happier with it then. Now, nothing was OK. The food was bad; the "help" (her word) was slow; the bedding was skimpy. Thank goodness for a television in front of each bed mounted from the ceiling and with remote controls. But I didn't know any of it my first day. What I remember of that day is wanting only to stay still in the bed but being too afraid to sleep. Did they know who I was and the amount of care I needed? Had my pain medication arrived with me? Were the brace and its directions there? Where was my family? I was finally assured all was in order. My medications were there and entered on my chart. The brace was on a chair by my bed. My daughter taped the instructions to the wall next to my bed. My flowers and family picture were arranged in view. I got kisses and gentle hugs. I think I fell asleep with the call device in one hand and the nonworking television remote in the other.

I woke up as an aide was bringing me lunch. That was a problem. I couldn't use my right hand very well and couldn't really sit up. It seemed the tray was stacked high with an impossible amount of food. The aide helped me eat a bit of it and tried to turn on the television for me. Clearly, the remote wasn't working. She mumbled,

"A person who knows how to make these work will be in sometime this week." But she and I were too busy getting me fed, turned, and dealing with the catheter to be too concerned. Although the catheter was removed later that week, in those first few days it made my life easier, since getting up to go to the bathroom seemed as daunting as climbing a mountain.

I didn't have to wait for the person who knew about remotes because a good, take-charge kind of friend stopped by soon after I had arrived. She looked at the remote, called a store, gave them the model number, and demanded they look up the code and read it to her so she could properly program it. They did. She did. The remote worked, and I was saved from fearsome thoughts and an unhappy roommate by game shows and sitcoms. I also got a good dose of perspective. Sometime during that first week I heard the news that Hurricane Katrina had hit New Orleans. It was very sobering and reminded me that I was in much better shape than so many people caught up in that despairing situation.

I think that on the second day an aide attempted to get me up and into the brace. The doctor and physical therapists had said it was important for me to be sitting up and walking a little each day. However, the aide could not figure out how to get it on. No, she did not want to read the instructions, and the next assistant read them but couldn't translate them into action. I don't know whether it was good recall or just desperation on my part, but I was able to explain enough to them to get it on. When my daughter came, I asked her to show a couple of aides how it was really supposed to work since she had paid such close attention to all the care I received in the hospital. Just knowing she would stop by each day helped me feel safe and know that no matter what did or didn't happen, by the next day it would be straightened out.

The first week in rehab is blurry. I realized that when it came to the staff, just like anywhere some people know what they are expected to do and that is exactly what they do. Some people give 180 percent and can't imagine doing less. Some people do as little as possible. However, when they are dealing with people whose pains, health, and well being depend on them, the differences mean more. I learned in that first week who would actually give me a sponge bath and who would always delay or not show up. I could count on a few to be right on time with the right medication and others who just showed up when they were ready. Some actually seemed to have read my chart and knew the type of care I needed and when. Others responded well if I told them, and a few were just unhappy to be bothered. The worst were those who knew they had power and seemed to genuinely enjoy abusing it. I only recall one, but what a difference she made to so many of us.

There was a time when I think my daughter let most of my friends know they should wait a few days to visit until I became stabilized. This plan was good for many reasons, mainly because as I started to become more aware of where I was and what was going on, I became more aware of my body, too. When the catheter was removed, I realized I felt like throwing up a lot and couldn't actually remember when I last had a bowel movement. I don't think I did in the hospital, even though I finally told the nurses I might have, and certainly not since moving to rehab. What an extremely painful ordeal that was. Even with every imaginable type of constipation medication, it still took more time to restore me to bowel health. Even years later I wouldn't dream of not having some roughage every day. I definitely don't want to go through that ever again. Fortunately for her, my unhappy roommate had checked out just prior to those days and a new roommate didn't appear until I was in better shape.

By the end of my first week I could use my right hand a little, was in my brace sitting in a wheelchair with a tray at mealtime, and wheeled through the halls. I saw where the physical therapy area was and knew I soon would be going there by a combination of wheelchair and walker. My doctor also sent the representative of a magnetic belt to fit me for one. It didn't take long and was reported to help bones heal faster. I didn't wear it all the time but followed the directions as well as possible. I felt ready to see friends and could focus on conversations.

As visitors came I also became more conscious of myself. Most of the swelling and bloating were gone. I made sure my hair was combed, and I at least had a robe on. But there was the problem of not having shaved my legs for at least three weeks. I know no one who came to see me was concerned with my legs, but I had enough vanity (not such a bad thing to have considering what I had been through) to want them looking more ladylike again. I was helpless to do anything. Because my legs were somewhat swollen and I had very little feeling in them, shaving seemed hazardous. My daughter bought a large tube of depilatory and lathered up a leg. What an amazing mess that was and disgusting to see as well. I consider her efforts at applying the goo, wiping it off, and rinsing each leg a pure act of love. To me it was a real morale booster.

Progress in stamina, movement, and good spirits kept me going. Therapy every day was so helpful in literally getting me back on my feet. When I started physical therapy, the therapist pushed my wheelchair close behind me while I used the walker for as far as I could go before becoming exhausted. I was able to get only half-way down my hall, and it seemed my walker and I would never be able to make it the many miles to the physical therapy room. Three weeks later I could easily go with the walker and realized it was only a short distance from my room. We started leg lifts with one-pound weights and moved to heavier ones. Nearby were three steps, and I was told I would be able to go up and down them by the time I went home.

I also had occupational therapy, which I thought was related to what I do at work! I found out it's therapy to prepare for all the everyday activities that occupy a normal life. Simple things like raising arms up to open a microwave oven and remove something or turn on a water faucet are new territory when movement is so limited.

I also had a small amount of improvement in my voice. It felt a little stronger and didn't fade as quickly.

I knew my surgery was unusual, but I didn't realize it also made me an unusual patient to the rehab staff. After a week of therapies I was experiencing pain, and I remembered the doctor telling me I would feel challenged but shouldn't do anything that caused pain. I told the therapists, but they reassured me the exercises were very minimal and my doctor wanted me to have therapy. Even their version of minimal was too much and some stitches broke, causing an extra trip to the doctor, fear of infection, and more time to be spent in the nursing home. I was both startled and frightened the morning I saw blood on my sheets from the incision. The doctor was upset that the therapists had pushed me too hard. The therapists were upset because the doctor hadn't provided detailed enough direction on exercise. I was just glad I had spoken up and was reminded that it's often better to listen to my body than to the experts.

We had to continue with the therapies and I wanted to because it meant I would be less helpless. It was ironic for someone as independent as I had always viewed myself to suddenly be so helpless. I thought I had come to terms with a loss of pride and ability to ask for help when needed, but that was nothing compared to the first two or three weeks after surgery.

To have the awareness of being extraordinarily fragile and that dire consequences could come from any number of movements was especially terrifying because I knew many people assisting me did not know the degree of my needs. To know I needed to be turned every two hours and lean on pillows caused a lot of stress about falling asleep. What would happen if no one came in to turn me? Although I had been assured it was temporary most of the time, I didn't know how long *temporary* would be or if I would fall into the *most of the time* category. The ventilator tube had damaged my vocal chords, and I couldn't speak loudly enough to call for help or get anyone's attention. My left leg was shaky and my right hand worked very haphazardly, still mostly numb from nerve reconnections. To be that helpless and not get lost in anger, bitterness, or despair required accepting at least some sense of it all being part of an adventure, just a part of the traveling and not the destination. It couldn't be a summation of what makes me who I am.

There were saving graces. Having visitors was so important; one reason was that I had too much time to get caught up in self-absorption but was aware they came to see the me they knew, the me I was still inside and was trying to unite with the physically recovering me. I knew they would listen if I was afraid and needed help. I felt the difference it made in me to be sure my hair was combed and that I looked presentable. However, I was not thinking just about me; I listened and looked at these people, seeing them and hearing what was going on in their lives and thoughts. I thought and responded and laughed and felt like a more complete human being than when I was just lying in bed or sitting in my wheelchair watching television.

About four weeks after the surgeries, some friends came to visit. They brought cookies and beverages, and we used a small dining area so we could have a little party. They walked patiently with me as I used all my energy to get to that room using my walker, not the wheelchair. The laughter and kindness, the reminders of happy times and friendship hit me hard; I started to cry and couldn't stop. I realized it was the first time since the surgery I had really allowed myself to feel my emotions, and the first crying I had done in probably a year. What a relief to get all that out of my system, especially in the company of friends.

The helplessness diminished as I progressed through a gentler set of physical and occupational therapies. I was able to use my walker to get to the physical therapy room, do the exercises, and return to my room. I was exhausted, but it was real, measurable progress. Each day I marveled at how short a distance it really was. Learning to use stairs came next, important because at my house my bedroom and the bathrooms with bathtubs and showers are upstairs. I knew I wouldn't be able to do all those stairs when I first got home, but I wanted to know the correct way to approach stairs and get a good start on them.

In occupational therapy we worked on the plan for my kitchen and dining room. How would I reach food and plates? Could I reach the microwave oven? How would I get food from the kitchen to the dining room and still use my walker? Then there was the matter of getting out of bed and getting dressed. I became adept at the side roll in and out of bed. I got a bra that closed in the front. Therapists showed me how to use tools to pull on my pants, socks, and shoes. Even more difficult was learning to take them off. For a while I put away all garments that had to be pulled over my head, and elastic drawstring pants became my friend. I got used to washing my face with a washcloth rather than bending over the sink. As I sat patiently being showered and having my hair washed, I was introduced to the curved, scrubby bath brush to reach all those areas I couldn't bend or stretch to reach, and I knew I would need help with the hair washing for a while. I also practiced with tools to grab objects at a distance, for assisting with shoes and socks as well as basic dressing. The tools are really ingenious, simple, and after some practice and patience easy to use. I can't stress enough how helpful the therapy proved to be when I got home and needed to be more self-sufficient. It was as important to my self-esteem and morale as it was for actual everyday living.

My daughter picked me up early one afternoon, and she carefully drove to her house. Getting into the car took creativity. I couldn't step into their SUV. Their other car had bucket seats that I would never have been able to get out of. We measured the size of the steps I was learning to use in physical therapy, and she found a child's step stool that was the same height. She helped me take that step, and I practiced backing into the seat as I had been shown in occupational therapy. Then I needed only a little assistance to move my legs and torso to face forward. A thin pillow wrapped in a plastic bag placed on the seat made turning or sliding into position much easier. All this equipment was necessary because I had been deeply cut from both the front and back, from lower abdomen and tailbone to my armpits. My muscles and nerves were still not up to the task of moving me. I felt exhilaration, emotion, and relief to be riding in a car for the five-minute ride to my daughter's house and to have a chance to visit with my granddaughter and son-in-law. I reflected on how different this visit was from all my prior visits and how differently I now viewed my life's activities.

I had my brace on and moved very slowly, aware there was the step stool to use getting out of the car. It surprised me that the downward steps were more difficult than stepping up. Apparently, stepping down used a different set of muscle groups I had never thought of before. In fact, every little thing required thought, attention, and energy. Prior to the surgery, I hadn't realized just how much I navigated through my days on automatic pilot. I never questioned my ability to take an item from the microwave oven, take a deep breath, or roll over and stretch in bed. I thought the limitation that pain had brought in the months prior to surgery had given me a hint of the recovery process, but recovery post surgery was a completely different situation.

Still, it was wonderful to be in a real home again. The living room was warm and family lived-in, such a contrast to the blandness of rehab. The family dog was excited to see me, but I couldn't really bend over to pet him and was too fragile for him to jump up on my lap. But I talked to him, and that was pleasing, too. We found a chair with a straight back, padded seat, and armrests I could sit in. My almost-two-year-old granddaughter bounded into the room and was completely enthralled with all my gadgets. The brace, the walker, even my purse were marvels to be touched and poked and played with. At first she wanted me to get down on the floor to play or pick her up. The wonderful thing about small children is their ability to accept differences. When she saw I couldn't do those things, she simply improvised ways around them to interact. It was also wonderful to see my son-in-law and hear him talk about work and the yard, all the things that make up real life.

I don't think I was there for more than twenty minutes when fatigue started to make everything—sitting, talking, listening—difficult. My daughter noticed, and when she asked if I were tired, I eagerly responded with, "Yes; all I can really think about is lying down." I was carefully helped back into the car, to my rehab room and my bed. I think my excursion had lasted less than an hour. I was so exhausted I couldn't move and didn't want to for the next few hours. I could see regaining stamina would be a big issue to deal with when I went home.

While I was at the doctor's office to remove the twenty-two large staples in my back, his nurse showed me how to take the brace on and off by myself. Doing it myself was very liberating.

My days at rehab filled with routine. I was wakened early with an aide handing me a washcloth to wipe my face and a breakfast tray arriving—usually in that order. Now that I could handle the brace by myself, I was able to get up to go the bathroom and get up with the walker to sit in my wheelchair for breakfast on my own. Next came a rest, then washing and dressing for physical therapy. Lunch, occupational therapy, a nap, and visitors were followed by dinner and my daughter dropping by. The evening was for television, music, and a crossword puzzle, if I was still awake. Talking on the phone was for urgent matters only since I couldn't really turn to get to the phone easily and my voice still tended to fail me regularly.

The doctor said that when I was able to walk up and down the three stairs in physical therapy, I could go home. I had very mixed feelings about going home. Of course I told everyone how excited I would be to go back to my own place and again have a sense of autonomy. I was excited but also frightened. The unknown immediate future held concerns. How would we be able to adjust the house to my many needs? How would we know what to do, and who would make the changes? At least I had made a good insurance decision. Without realizing it at the time, one of my smartest moves after starting my job was to read about all my benefit options. I checked *yes* in the box for long-term disability insurance, only a few dollars extra a month. Recovery was difficult enough. Without it and my regular health insurance, I would have had so much more stress and difficulty. Even more humbling was the knowledge that if I hadn't had insurance, I might have wound up in a wheelchair on disability without the option to try any other way.

Meanwhile, friends and coworkers wanted to know how I was doing. I certainly wasn't up to so many questions or even the well-wishers. My family was overloaded assisting me while trying to go on with their lives. We didn't want to leave updated voice mails for any caller to pick up. My daughter set up a blog and diligently updated information on my condition. Friends responded, and she read their messages to me when she came to visit. I can't express how wonderful it was to hear those messages. To have a single, simple way to let everyone know how I was doing was a lifesaver for my family as well. My daughter also included information regarding when I could have visitors and where the rehabilitation center was located. She later added a section regarding help I needed or would need so people could sign up.

When we set up the page, we called it "Carol's Adventure," and it had a color photo of a Chinese teahouse in a garden. It started with the introduction I had written in early August:

> Here's an opportunity for my friends to share the upcoming adventure I'm about to have, called "Life as a Metal Sculpture." The sculpting begins the morning of August 15 and continues via surgery through the 17th. I will be at Hospital X. If you want to know how I'm doing, this blog will be updated regularly. If you want to know what you can do to help, please direct your prayers to reflect, "May the surgeons perform flawlessly; may complications be minimal; may recovery be swift, with God's grace."

Later in my recovery, I will need more assistance in the form of phone calls, grocery shopping, etc. This blog will also be a source for requests and scheduling.

After August 15, page 2 will contain details on my progress. The countdown to surgery begins by being sure to celebrate every day. Each one is a jewel. I invite you to join me in laughing, enjoying each other's company, and feeling generally happy to be breathing and alive on this planet.

Here is a sample of the messages my daughter wrote for my friends:

8/15 – 8:30am went into surgery. Expected surgery time is five hours, followed by recovery and then ICU.

8/16 – Carol is doing great. Getting sleep and resting up for the next surgery. Tomorrow's surgery will begin at 7:30AM and could take up to 10 hours. Please keep praying. It works!

8/17– Carol's second surgery went great. Everything went smooth and quicker than expected. See, your prayers did it! She is recovering in ICU tonight and on a ventilator. As you can imagine, this is a time when she needs lots of rest. If you would like to email me (her daughter) a message to read to her, please send it to [her email address]. We prefer that she not have visitors while in ICU but you can send her your love and thoughts via email.

9/24 – A great day. Carol came over to my house for about 1 1/2 hours. A nice break from the routine and a good chance for her to see the family. I took her back once she started to get tired. We plan another trip out tomorrow late afternoon. She is feeling strong and ready to go home. So now it is a matter of coordinating everything. Hoping for Tuesday. Will keep you posted.

10/2 & 3 – Carol is doing great but is surprised everyday by how quickly she gets tired. Even visiting with a friend is exhausting. Please email me if you want to call or visit Carol and I'll see if she is up for it, starting this weekend and next week.

10/16 – Hard to believe that it has only been two months since Carol had her surgeries. Her recovery has been amazing so far and looks to only continue to get better. As she continues to get strong, Carol can walk a little further each day and around the house without her walker quite a bit. At the end of October I will discontinue updating this website and Carol will start responding to calls and emails. Thanks to everyone for sending your love and support to Carol. It makes a difference. You make a difference.

The last entry is from me:

> As of November 14th this site will no longer be available. You can contact me directly at my home phone number or email address. More gratitude than I can express to all of you for your flowers, cards, visits, prayers and good thoughts. They have aided and continue to aid my recovery in amazing ways. You will remain in my prayers as well and I hope to be in communication with you all.

Carol R. Palo

We are the ones for whom we have been waiting.
—Hopi Elders

CHAPTER 5

RECLAIMING MYSELF

~⁀〜

*G*oing home sounds so great and so simple. If the doctor determines you are doing well enough now to go home, you can just get in the car and pick up your life where you left off. But that isn't the reality at all. I am grateful for all the questions I asked my doctor before surgery and for all the information from my insurance company as well.

Of course the wonderful thing about going home is having your own little corner of the earth where you call the shots. It turns out being able to decide if the music will be louder or softer and what you want to eat and when is a really big deal. Looking around and seeing those items that remind you of your values, your family, and what you like to look at and be around is reaffirming. It is also a milestone in the steps to independence, whatever that turns out to be.

For me, there was also the matter of getting around. My bedroom was upstairs and, when I first arrived home, too many stairs to climb. My bed was incredibly comfortable, but it didn't have the adjustments to lower or raise the head or the entire bed. A hospital bed was necessary for a while and it would be parked in the living room. A half bath on the first floor was great for a quick wash up and basic needs. Even if I'd had a full bathroom on the main floor I wouldn't have been able to take a bath, nor had I the balance and strength for a shower. I required an aide twice a week so I could have a sponge bath and my hair washed. A nurse needed to come every other day to check and refresh the dressing on my torn sutures. An occupational therapist and physical therapist were scheduled as well. I was lucky enough to have my son stay at the house for the first few weeks. Answering the door for everyone and trying to fix a meal or change sheets were just too much for me when I first got home.

My house needed some handicap-friendly adjustments as well. Being willing to ask for help was so important. I was surprised how many people were willing to lend a hand, but they weren't mind readers. I had friends, as it turned out, with carpentry skills. When my daughter pulled the car into the garage and I got out, it was the first time I really noticed there was a step up from the garage to the house. It looked like a very big step. How fortunate that my carpenter friends put up a little grab bar for me to hold on to. I really needed it. They also added a second railing to my inside stairs so I had a railing on each side. As I learned to navigate those steps, having a railing on each side to hold with both hands made the process so much easier. Later I saw they had installed a shower bar just outside my large shower stall and a handheld showerhead inside, which made showering while I sat possible.

While I was in the rehabilitation center, my daughter and I pored over catalogs, trying to determine which of the many types of shower chairs or stools, walkers, aids for reaching, and a seemingly endless variety of possible tools to purchase. The occupational therapist gave us good tips on tools and supplies. Once again my insurance company directed us to its supplier of choice, which streamlined the process. We needed to purchase some items. Other items, including the hospital bed, could be rented by the month. Some items were covered by insurance and some weren't. Some were available at a regular variety store. Having occupational therapy before coming home was helpful in several ways. I had the chance to try a couple of shower benches or chairs, different types of long-handled bath brushes, and an incredible array of toilet enhancers that raised the seat to a more comfortable level. Learning how to use many of the strange new devices for putting on and taking off socks, shoes, and pants helped determine which ones I should purchase.

The day I came home was crazy. What a job of coordination it was for my family. We knew a truck was scheduled to deliver the hospital bed and set it up around the same time I was to arrive home. The same truck might have the toilet accommodations, two walkers (one for upstairs and one for downstairs), and a cane, although those items might come separately. We all needed to be available when the delivery people gave instructions on how to adjust all the equipment to fit my needs. I arrived home exhausted from the drive and needing the bed *now*, with concerns about needing the toilet and its new attachments soon. Thank goodness a friend was handy to direct traffic and get instructions. Getting me home and settled in was definitely a team effort, but there was a wild card in all of it. The morning I was to return home, my son discovered a very active wasp nest in the eaves of my front porch. Fortunately, an exterminator rushed over and removed it just before I got home. It would have been daunting to dodge angry wasps as equipment, family, and I all arrived.

As I write this account, it is strangely interesting to look back through my notes and memories at the "me" I was at that time. I marvel at the messages and updates my daughter left for friends and coworkers after the surgeries and during my early weeks in rehab. She was always so gracious and upbeat in her telling of the day's activities and accomplishments, and so able to minimize the sometimes traumatic and painful situations. As I read through her comments, they reminded me of some important lessons learned.

April's accounting of the surgery and the days directly after were as accurate as anything I could come up with. I remember at least some of the people who visited me, and seeing and feeling them there was really important to me even if I wasn't able to let anyone know. Not being able to move much made having the beautiful flowers placed in my range of vision important. When I looked at them I saw beauty and knew I was remembered and cared about. When people take the time to show they care, it really matters.

When we were planning to leave the hospital for rehab, I heard there were two options. I could go in a wheelchair in a cab designed to transport wheelchairs, or I could go by ambulance. The insurance would pay either, depending on what my doctor recommended. Thank goodness we asked all these questions about transportation, because I don't know if they would have been brought up otherwise. I heard some of the staff voice surprise and what I thought was a bit of derision because I was opting for the ambulance. My doctor agreed it was warranted and would create less physical stress for me, and he was right. Even with extra drugs, my daughter next to me talking and holding my hand, and a very slow and gentle ride, it was still excruciating and exhausting. I can't imagine keeping a tough-gal image would ever have been worth sucking it up and riding in a cab.

My daughter wrote about getting into a routine during those first few days at rehab. The thing about being quite helpless and knowing it is that you become creative in finding any little things to help you feel empowered or in control of something. One of those I found empowering was the remote control to the television. I could escape my little temporary world and move into game shows, the news, travel shows, most anything that helped pass the difficult and frightening moments of reality in the first days there.

There was the realization that I was dependent in every conceivable way on people who were just showing up to do their job. Some aides and staff were cheerful and genuinely helpful and some were not. It didn't take me long to determine that I could make a big difference in how well I felt and how much I improved by being as involved in what was happening to me as possible. Moaning, complaining, or getting angry were just wastes of my precious time and energy. Another empowering tool was keeping a log of when I got medications, when I had been turned, and which days I had showers. This activity helped me regain the use of my right hand; it was a form of physical therapy. It was hard for me to write and it came slowly, but I had time. It also grounded me in looking out for myself and offered a reality check. Within a few weeks, the aides relied on me to remind them of when I got my next medication, and which one. I was able to push the button for assistance and say with sureness it was time to help me turn to the other side. I could show anyone the notes tracking the times. It reassured me that my mind was still sharp enough to be useful to me.

I remembered what it had felt like to take nothing for granted—breathing without pain or the surety that what I thought would come out of my mouth actually would, to know every movement my body was able to make. How wonderful it felt now to have the freedom to move with minimal pain and to feel the outdoors, the sun and breeze on my skin.

I think of practicing getting in and out of a car using a step stool so I could visit my daughter's home and then think ahead to going to my home. It was amazing how a life I lived as my birthright seemed so far away, as if it had happened in another lifetime, not in the same calendar year. That short car ride to visit family was a reminder of trees, cars, real-life activity, and a pace of life happening that wasn't experienced in nursing home scenarios. We had real conversations not related to my back issues. How exhausting but wonderful.

Coming home and starting the next phase of my journey was exciting because it was a step toward getting my life back, but it was also worrisome. As intrusive as always being watched and told what to do was, the thought of life with no trained personnel around 24/7 was hard to imagine. I reassured myself with the reality of not really being alone. One day at a time, healing progressively, I believed I would become much healthier and happier. It's OK to be afraid; I just needed to remind myself I didn't have to live in the fear but focus on happier possibilities.

I ran into an old friend recently. She is a retired surgical nurse who had been through some surgeries of her own. We caught up with what we had each been doing in the years since my surgery. She remembered how emphatic I had been about not needing a hospital bed in my living room. I was sure I could go upstairs and would want to sleep in my own wonderful bed, and how sure I had been that the stairs would be no issue; after all, I had a hand rail to hold on to. She said that every suggestion she made that I might need to look at in my day-to-day activities I had scoffed at—the idea that I would be so dependent and fragile. It reminds me how frightening the prospect of having the surgery was, let alone any possible changes to my lifestyle, even temporary ones. Of course she was right. It was just incomprehensible to understand how the smallest motion at the wrong angle, or a chair that was a little too tilted, tall, or curved could make the difference between agony and some comfort. Even in those last months before surgery, I had become an expert in chair angles, padding, and how much pain would be involved in walking on various types of floor coverings.

It felt wonderful to finally lie down in the hospital bed in my own home and rest. Not being on someone else's schedule was heaven. To be able to eat when I wanted and sleep without being interrupted by staff or people moaning was almost immediately restorative. I was able to cut back on medication when I was able to think about when I really needed them versus having someone bringing them and taking them per a schedule. I felt safe knowing I didn't have to worry about food, laundry, the phone ringing, or much else with my son there. His presence was such a blessing. My daughter had taken over my financial responsibilities. Because I knew the surgery was coming, I was able to set aside money to prepay most of my monthly bills. I also signed several checks for her to fill in if she needed them.

It wasn't long before a lifestyle routine fell into place. Once, when the visiting nurse came to check and change the dressing from opened stitches on my back, she implied that she would not come back and treat me if I didn't sign paperwork she had with her that claimed I would be responsible for payment if my insurance company didn't pay. Of course the care providers need to be paid, but to threaten a patient who just came home and is medicated seemed unethical to me. The fact that I signed the papers shows I was not my normal self. Looking back, I wonder if medications made me feel more threatened than what was actually happening. Regardless, my back healed quickly and soon there was no need for the nurse. I remember telling someone about the situation, and the response was that I should report it. But honestly, I had my hands full with healing physically, physical therapy, just breathing, and, of course, more forms and phone calls with the insurance company than I could deal with. I had no energy to pursue my thoughts on that nurse's way of dealing with patients. My son took on a lot of the insurance matters, so between us issues were resolved and payments were made. It seemed at times that dealing with what was covered by whom and under what conditions with verifications was almost harder to deal with than the surgery. I think that is probably typical. It is due diligence, making sure the dollars and processes are in order.

The physical therapist came three times a week, and we worked on adding stairs, one at a time, along with balance and planning to actually get out of the house. I felt very shaky on my feet. Even though there were just two steps between me and the sidewalk, it seemed overwhelming. Again I found that going up stairs and down stairs took different sets of muscles; going down, for some reason, really threw me off. We compromised by going out the garage door at the back of the house to the alley. As the door opened, I was horrified by what appeared to be a very long, steep driveway making its way to the alley. I looked at it many times later and wondered how a very short and gently, barely graded downward slope could have been so daunting. But my brain saw only that there was no flat easy surface but instead something different to cope with. With the therapist near me and a death grip on my walker, I edged toward the nice, flat alley. I was both elated and exhausted after arriving at its familiar flatness.

The most helpful thought throughout all the therapy was noting that I was in the process of recovery. I didn't know what that final product would be like, but I knew my current situation was not the new normal, and I was very grateful for that. It wasn't long before I was walking to the end of the block with my walker, even using the front steps. The next goal was transferring from the walker to a cane. Eventually the physical therapist came just twice a week. At that point I no longer needed to have a chair on the landing halfway up the staircase; I could pause to catch my breath and continue up to the second floor. The second floor was a milestone. It meant I would soon be able to sleep in my own bed and relearn how to take a shower on my own.

I was able to use the little half bath on the main floor to wash up and brush my teeth. It had barely enough room to maneuver the walker, but it was workable. The value of having a home visit with an occupational therapist made the early weeks of being at home much simpler. During that visit we walked from room to room and measured and imagined every movement that goes into the basics of everyday living. Her tips and reality checks were priceless, little things like would the walker fit in the bathroom and if so at what angle; if not, was there something I could hold on to for balance or would a cane work better. One of the most luxurious feelings I experienced was having a home care attendant come twice a week to wash my hair and give me a sponge bath during the time I was unable to go upstairs and shower.

Healing took up a tremendous amount of energy. I often found the process of consuming food, deciding what to pick up on my fork, trying to get the still numb right hand to work, and the hard work of actually chewing the food really tired me out, making a few bites feel like a full-time job. I look back and realize a lot of progress really was being made quite rapidly.

A few months before surgery, a good friend gave me one of the most practical and helpful tips I could imagine. She said, "Realistically, who do you know that could really turn their whole life off and just be there for you and the minutia of your daily needs? The answer is really not anyone. But to call not only friends but acquaintances and neighbors with a one time or twice a month request to pick up my mail? Or would they stop by and visit and do a load of laundry? Could they come by once in the next couple of weeks and bring me some groceries; I have a list and cash?" Yes, it turned out that lots of people were very willing to do just one simple thing at a time and in a way that worked for them and their lives. In the beginning my daughter orchestrated it all; eventually I was able to take it over. We installed a lockbox on my front porch containing my house key and gave the combination to those wonderful people who volunteered to assist me. I knew someone had to come at least twice a day for a while. I needed to wear elastic hosiery to prevent blood clots and swelling during the day, but I was unable to put them on or take them off. Someone came by and helped with the hosiery, chatting a little, seeing that I was eating, if I had clean clothing or was in need of groceries. Someone came by and did a load of laundry, perhaps after bringing in my mail. Whatever each person was able to do during a visit made a huge difference.

My daughter made arrangements to bring her laptop and worked from my house every Thursday. I had the foresight to have a router and wireless access installed throughout my house, which later made possible my reentry to work from my dining room table.

My energy slowly came back. I also got to the point when the physical therapist stopped coming by to walk with me. I had made it to the mailbox with the walker and even bought a basket and pouch to attach for carrying the mail and other loose items. I did graduate to a cane by the time I had friends accompany me on walks around the block. But what would I do when I had to make those walks by myself? What if I fell? I read a book on mindful walking, and it gave me the confidence to walk looking straight ahead, not down at my feet. It is also what a physical therapist said to do, but I needed reinforcement to actually do it. I came to believe that if I focused only on looking ahead and let each foot take the next right step I would be OK. If I tripped and fell, I thought I would try to fall onto someone's lawn (rather than the sidewalk) and lay there until someone saw me and helped me up. Since most people in my neighborhood worked during the day I knew it might be a long time, so I really focused on being involved in nothing but the walk. I did not fall.

Halloween came and I wanted to greet and hand out candy to the trick or treaters. I knew many neighbors had small children and really looked at the opportunity as a fun activity in a sea of serious actions. A friend bought bags of candy and left my porch light on. I answered the door in my huge brace, the boxy magnetic belt and a gag arrow through my head. I had a better costume than most of the trick or treaters, and some of the little kids' eyes got as big as saucers when I opened the door. After an hour or so I had to stop. Too much up and down and conversation for one evening, but it was fun to step out of my spine-focused world and be a part of the neighborhood activities.

With the beginning of November, at about three months after surgery, also came my promise of working part time from home. I had my laptop set up at the dining room table, and although my right hand was still mostly numb, I was doing personal emails for a few minutes each day. Now as a starting point I had to think about how work would flow and how much I could do. I don't remember exactly how we set it up, but I think I agreed to two hours a day five days a week just checking email, changing to three hours a day sometime in early December. Both my work phone and email were disabled from taking messages and referred contacts to people who had taken over my duties. My ability to speak had improved, but I thought it better to wait with phone calls until I was more sure how I would sound. Also, I had been out of the whole workplace loop and was totally focused on me and my back, hospital, doctors, rehab center, and my quiet home; I needed some time to transition back into a work frame of mind. I remember having my computer reset to accept emails, and did they come! Those first couple of weeks were spent reading and assessing what had been going on, what needed to be done, what changes had occurred. I had let go of my job completely with all it entailed and was glad to be starting off slowly.

Next, voice mail was activated and I started working more fully from home. I think the activity helped my hand gain function and also kept my mind a little more agile. I treasured those Thursdays that my daughter came over. Although we both worked at the dining room table (me more napping and less actual work), just having her there and being able to talk and get her assistance at breaks and lunch added a wonderful dimension to our relationship.

My son came back for Thanksgiving, and we celebrated at my daughter and son-in-law's home. My mother was also picked up from the assisted living facility where she lived. I had not yet seen her, knowing it would be distressing for her to see me so thin and pale and in the massive brace and belt. But it was a major holiday. I knew I was getting better and hoped that the next time I saw her, I'd be looking more normal. Besides, families deal with whatever life presents as best they can, and we did, too. Of course my mom was upset to see me as I was, and because of her deteriorating memory mentioned her concern every few minutes. The saving grace of the memory issue was that it also kept her from realizing how long it had been since she had actually seen me. For me, stepping back into real family color, sounds, chaos, food, smells, and pets was so restorative, even though it took enormous energy just to be present.

My granddaughter was almost three years old at that time and brought such a different and healthier perspective as she naturally accepted my mom in her wheelchair, me in the strange large brace, and our inability to move around much. She was curious about it all, but clearly loved us, taking both of us as part of her cherished family regardless of the differences we presented. It is a gift to be treated as more than the wheelchair, walker, or handicap.

It was also wonderful to have my son back for that week. He took me, with my walker, in the car for a little excursion. We went to a restaurant and some shops. I was thinking about the upcoming holidays, and although I could shop online, and did most of my shopping that year online, what I really missed was touching things. Being able to go somewhere and touch the fabric or feel the weight and sense of it turned out to be a more important part of the shopping experience than I had ever thought. The human capacity to take for granted really came home to me every time I bumped into something simple and basic that I had never much thought of before, like being in a store and waiting in a cashier's line to buy something, or wandering through the aisles without worry of being bumped into. At first I went out with the walker for extra stability, not just for my own balance issues but because so many people are busy with their own thoughts and moving quickly that being bumped into was a real possibility. The walker stood out more than a cane would have, although my son was so protective I was more worried about what he might do to someone who ran into me than I was of being bumped!

The bag for mail attached to my walker worked well except when my orders of holiday gifts arrived. All the mailboxes on my street were joined together with large package receptacles below that could be opened with a key. I couldn't bend to reach those boxes, and even if I could, I was on doctor's orders not to lift anything more than five pounds. Fortunately, several people were in the habit of picking up their mail shortly after the time the mail usually arrived, so I would wait for someone to come by and asked for assistance. Sometimes I needed someone to carry the package to my house as well, and no one ever turned me down. I remember hoping that when I was healthier I would remember and help others.

Becoming more self-sufficient as it became more and more possible was satisfying beyond words. Each time it chipped away at the fear of never being whole again. I think in the early days of my recovery being whole meant that my life experience would be as close as possible to what it was prior to the spinal disability. Today, I think of *whole* as however a person chooses to define it.

Part of my recovery was walking every day, outside if at all possible, which meant coming to terms with the fear that if I fell I would be alone and dependent on whoever might be available to assist me, as well as the possibility of injury. Except for getting my mail, I used the cane for these walks. At some point, with the physical therapist's OK, I had to say I would always either use a cane or start moving toward walking on my own. All the way through the ordeal it helped me to realize I was responsible for making these choices. Whatever they were, I would be the one living with them.

In mentioning possible injury, I realize I've said nothing yet about pain. Some comments on pain and medication are necessary because the issue comes up for anyone who is facing major pain. Prior to surgery my doctor told me I would need all my energy to be focused on healing, that being in pain would slow and hamper my recovery. I had serious concerns about the addictive nature of many medications and discussed them in detail with him. I think because he was knowledgeable about medications and I was very honest and specific with him, we were able to come up with a workable plan. He promised that if I followed his directions always and completely, I would have minimal pain and emerge with just an occasional need for Tylenol. It proved to be true. We moved from morphine in the hospital to Oxycontin and Vicodin. Then, toward the end of December, he said it was time to take just Tylenol. It seemed to have come too quickly, and I reminded him of concerns about pain. He reminded me that I had agreed to follow his instruction. I cut back on the medications, and in a few weeks I was taking only two or three Tylenols a day. It really amazed me. I had not been in unendurable pain the whole time, and I believe that spiritual assistance played as great a role as my wise doctor's plan.

What I learned about Oxycontin is its ability to seduce us into thinking the drug has no hold on us. Here's how I would describe it: Imagine you are going out with friends on a sunny day and you have no sunglasses. A friend loans you hers, and they have a nice yellow tint. Everything looks great, and the sun doesn't bother your eyes. A few days later you are going out with other friends. Again you need to borrow sunglasses. This friend has normally tinted sunglasses. You feel disappointed. Yes, the sun is not bothering your eyes, but the great tint that makes everything a little better is gone. That is what Oxycontin felt like to me— just a nice sunny glow to everything. No wonder it is so psychologically addictive, let alone what it may be doing physically.

Just prior to the Christmas holidays, I was able to go for a walk and work three hours each day. I also started to participate in conference call meetings. I even had enough energy for my final occupational therapy: up and down my stairs, return to my own bed, and have a Christmas tree rather than a hospital bed in my living room. I would be taught to take a shower by myself. Life was good.

Christmas and my granddaughter's birthday brought me out of my house and to my daughter's much-decorated and festive home. When I wrote about those times, I thought I would remember such happy events in great detail because so much of my life was made of recovery's mundane activities. However, I found I didn't remember anything. Even more startling to me was that my son, son-in-law, and daughter didn't remember anything of that holiday season, either. I think this highlights how easy it is to minimize the stress and trauma to everyone involved in long, serious medical situations. The energy it takes can simply and quietly overwhelm most everything, even the joys.

A new year began. More than four months had gone by since my surgery. I was so grateful to have the surgery behind me. A friend came over and walked through my house with me, looking at all the areas either too low or too high for me to access, and I didn't yet know when or if I would be able to make use of them. She helped rearrange items to suit my needs and abilities. Being able to reach for something without always bumping into *I can't do this either* really helped me to feel capable and valuable to myself. It's interesting that in a society in which what you do is so intrinsic to your value, simply being me did not seem quite worthy enough in itself. I learned to modify old habits, like washing dishes by hand slowly and placing on a rack to dry. I then left them there until I needed them again. In the past I used the dishwasher, but now I couldn't bend to put dishes in or take them out. I also had been thorough about putting everything away in the cupboards or drawers, but now that just meant extra and difficult work. I had tools and received training on how to use them as part of occupational therapy. I didn't want to use the tools, but in those early months they were my key to independence. They enabled me to put on my socks and slippers and take them off. I was able to reach so much more with the grabber tools. Just having a raised toilet seat sitting on top of my regular one in both bathrooms allowed me to use them without needing assistance getting up. Yes, every little thing required a new look and action.

I saw continual improvement in my abilities to move, think, adapt, and be free of the serious medications. I was amazed at how far I had come in four-plus months, but I couldn't really look at how much was still to be done. I equated good recovery with my expectations that I would return to work and have less dependence on the help of others. It was still hard for me to imagine what that would be like.

By late January I knew I had to come up with a plan for return-ing to the office, and that also involved how I would get there since it was a fifteen-mile commute each way. I had felt like a contributing member of my workplace by working several half-days each week from home. It was time to try a few hours at the office. My son came for a timely visit and drove me there. I was both excited and nervous. I still wore the cumbersome brace and moved slowly. My right hand was not yet completely normal—it can take a long time for nerves to heal. Fortunately, he had brought his computer and stayed at the office with me. I had hoped to stay several hours and leave still feel-ing reasonably refreshed, but I didn't realize how very different being in the workplace is from working at home. The tempo was very fast paced. People moved and spoke quickly, and they expected the same from me. Reaching for the computer and phone was exhausting and painful. After two hours I was so tired and with such pain that it was a real effort to get back to the car. I couldn't get home fast enough to lie down and just rest. It was a very sobering reality check of how long it might be before I could go into work and have normal days. I feared that might be too much to aspire to. Still, it was important to put in the appearance just to claim my office and show that I am still doing the job and not going anywhere. I've found that if you want to claim your seat in any area of your life, you have to take the action. That is what I did.

When I got home and settled in, I pulled out the calendar and thought about how I could phase back in to working at the office. The reality was that a great deal of the early spring projects entailed heavy computer work and conference calls, which I could easily still do from home. The lack of energy I experienced at that first visit became the incentive to work all the harder in physical therapy for agility and strength, which meant walking more, especially the stairs, and doing more reaching and light lifting in my daily activities. I explained to my boss and work group that I would do the computer work from home through February, then in March would start coming in one day a week to handle the areas that required me to be on site. Someone at work and generous friends assisted me with the commute.

In February I started getting in and out of my car, practicing the moves needed to drive, and backing the car out of and into the garage. Fortunately, I had a two-car garage so there was a lot of leeway for those maneuvers. Not being able to twist my body to look behind was intimidating, and I needed a lot of practice. I tried some specialty mirror placements, but they were confusing; adjusting just the side and rear mirrors worked pretty well. In early March I slowly drove around my quiet residential neighborhood, getting used to the movement and change.

In April I started driving to work. I began with two days a week and moved to three days a week by early May. All the activity was still exhausting, but because I had been accruing vacation time while working part time from home, I was able to take at least every other Friday off either as a whole or half day. That was a saving grace. By the time I hit the one-year-from-surgery mark, I was back to working full time.

Even harder than the physical restraints were the emotional and psychological adjustments. I had spent about eight months surrounded by friends, doctors, and therapists who were there for me and my welfare. They were caring and nurturing and kind. That is not what a busy workplace going through its whirling dervish pace of annual closing and balancing of budgets, profits, and such is like. I was back. There was a lot of work to be done—elbowing for next year's budgets, justifications for the past year's activities—and I was expected to step up to the plate and wade in like everyone else in management did. From April through June I went home and cried a lot as I came to terms with the pace.

I spent the following year fine tuning my new reality, which was still changing. I realized that a healing body takes the time it needs. The good news is the hope of continued progress it brings. In time I gained more comfort at work by getting stronger and faster as well as by making adjustments to my work space. Driving became easier, and I was able to start getting together with friends on weekends.

About one-and-a-half years after surgery, I attempted to travel again by visiting the friends in Palm Springs whom I had visited on my last trip prior to surgery. The trip was just a few days long, but it was quite wonderful not to need a wheelchair to get to the plane and to actually spend some time with them without lying down in pain. It was also a good indicator of both the great healing progress and how far I still was from the easygoing traveler I had once been. Most helpful was remembering that any ability was a gift of the surgery, my body's healing ability, and good therapy. I had vowed to take any victory available and run with it, and so I did.

My Life as a Metal Sculpture

Today I know there are unexpected bonuses of awareness, knowledge, and insights possible. I most likely wouldn't have had their benefit without going through the whole process of discovery through post-surgery, and I would have been the poorer for it.

Here are some things I learned:

- In many ways I am a more compassionate person with others and with myself.
- I don't take for granted the ability to move, even in the smallest ways.
- It's okay to still be careful about sitting. So what if I am sensitive to the too-hard seat, the seat angle, or a hard back that catches me in the wrong places. None of it comes even close to the degree it once was.
- Having limited physical ability on an ongoing basis is a challenge. For me it translates into no twisting or stretching of the back and some nerve and swelling problems in the feet.
- It is wonderful to be able to sleep freely in different positions. It is a smile-producing pleasure.
- It took time, but I found the ability to accept the people who said they couldn't stand by me or help in any way because of their own issues, without my being judgmental or resentful.
- I've acquired an understanding of what being very helpless feels like, even though it was for a short time. I think it requires every bit of courage, humility, and humor that anyone in such a situation can muster.

As I write, several years after the surgery, I am still grateful for its success. It is encouraging to feel how willing my body is to try and accommodate my requests. There is still not only progress but also the bumping into limitations that come from moving further and further into the world of action.

PART TWO
PERSPECTIVES

Take care of yourself—you never know when the world will need you.
—Rabbi Hillel

Chapter 6

Everyday Life

⁓

My Life as a Metal Sculpture was written to be of assistance to others with medical situations, not meant to be just the telling of my story. Unfortunately, my situation is not unique but only one of many stories about unexpected life situations. My experience has to do with a twisted spine, so that's what I wrote about. But I think much of what made up this journey is transferable to many medical difficulties. Regardless of the medical trauma, the impact affects both patients and everyone in their circle of living.

I wouldn't be who I am and my story would be vastly different without the assistance of family and friends. An accounting of my journey wouldn't be complete without their perspectives, comments, and remembrances. I think the effect on them is important and worth considering.

This section also includes the journeys of a few people who had to face and deal with their own versions of unwelcome medical situations. My hope is that it provides a broader view of how various crises and illnesses can be dealt with.

Unexpected serious medical situations can be life changing and certainly take up a huge amount of focus and energy. The nature of dealing with new and unwanted issues is absorbing. As if this isn't enough of a load, most of us don't live in a vacuum. The good news is that we are not alone. We are surrounded by coworkers, neighbors, friends, family, and even those people we don't know directly but interact with, such as other drivers on the road and cashiers in a store. The bad news is that we are not alone. Our attitude, actions, and day-to-day activities affect all of them.

I had a time of self-absorption while I came to terms with my new situation and a new way of thinking about myself and my routine. People I came into contact with didn't get my attention or concern as they would have under normal circumstances. I was impatient or distracted when shopping. When in conversations, my mind was often miles away. Eventually, I realized that my sense of comfort with other people was slipping away, and it was probably my doing.

I withdrew from contact with people at work and lost a lot of my sense of humor while I was in the trying-to-come-to-terms-with stage. I didn't want anyone to know what was going on with me, which left my coworkers wondering if I were mad at them and also set the scene for speculation about me. Later, when I started falling at work, it was evident something was physically wrong. By then I was comfortable letting them know about my back problems and that I was looking at several solutions. I had already, gradually, started cross-training a few people and sharing my information when I felt the timing was right.

I was cranky waiting in line at the grocery store because I was in pain. I'm also not a very patient person, which added to my crankiness. Many times I wanted to stop at the store on the way home from work but couldn't find a parking place without walking quite a way. That, combined with getting groceries and waiting in line, became just too much for me. A partial solution involved admitting I needed a handicap placard and going through my doctor to get the paperwork. He erased a lot of my denial regarding the need for handicapped status, was even surprised I had waited so long with my request. Parking closer to the store's entrance combined with my admitting "Sorry I'm having a difficult day" at the check stand made the situation better.

I became a little more compassionate toward my fellow drivers. I now realized from my own experience that wanting to rush somewhere wasn't everyone's priority. I had to really concentrate on ignoring pain and driving safely, even though that sometimes had me driving slower than I would have at one time.

Making these adjustments helped me to feel I was still a part of the everyday world in a way I had always taken for granted.

Be kinder than necessary, for everyone you meet is fighting some kind of battle.
—Author unknown

Chapter 7

Recollections and Tips

❧

Slowly I had become more and more isolated. I turned down invitations from friends to go out, giving the impression I was tired from work or had other plans. As my back problems accelerated, on work days it was all I could do to get home, grab a bite to eat, and make it upstairs. On weekends, when I had more time to lie down, my reality contained too much difficulty in figuring out where to stand or sit or just be, without adding more pain. I deprived myself of a lot of support and care until I was able to let go of my false pride and the fear that came every time I talked about it and felt what it meant.

Being able to share my situation with at least a few friends became critical. Without good, caring friends I might have spent a few nights lying on the floor by the stairs, unable to make it upstairs to bed or anywhere else. When the ice stopped working and the pain took over, it was also less traumatic to have friends take me to the emergency room rather than calling an ambulance.

Friends accompanied me out of state to see specialists. Taking their vacation days, they helped turn that time into adventures instead of difficult and dreaded situations.

I also had also the opportunity to practice acceptance and compassion with a few friends who, because of their situations, said they found my situation too traumatic for them to deal with. They wished me well, but I didn't hear from them until I contacted them much later.

When I first found out about my back situation, my family consisted of my mother, son, daughter, and son-in-law. My mother was starting to have severe memory problems, and I didn't tell her anything about my spinal issues. My granddaughter was still a gleam in her parents' eyes. When I first told the rest of my family about my back problems and a potential surgery, they appreciated knowing what was going on and hoped my back would get better. I don't think I went into the stark details or how terrifying it all felt. I was going to do everything I could to keep the doctor's prognosis from becoming a reality. At first I thought I might never need to tell them the details of that initial doctor visit. As time went by, it became necessary to move from me with my problems to a family team who would deal with the trauma certainly coming our way.

My Son, Nick

For several years before the surgery, the condition of my Mom's back had been degrading. At first, it seemed merely to limit the scope of some of her activities. However, it seemed to worsen at an exponentially quicker pace. By the time of her surgery, the pain and the limitations of her movements seemed to have moved the question of surgery from the realm of possibility to that of necessity.

I remember much more about the events surrounding her surgery than the progression of back issue more generally, perhaps because I was living out of state and visited Portland at most a handful of times a year. Mostly, I recall the all-too-common sadness and concern that comes with watching someone you love suffer while there is little or nothing you could do to address it.

Those concerns and fears are myriad and far too complex to articulate fully within this format. However, they certainly included the following issues. First, it was a radical surgery, one that, although more likely than not to succeed, carried with it substantial risks. That concern was mitigated by the knowledge that my Mom was experiencing intolerable pain and, absent the surgery, it would significantly worsen over time. Related to that concern was what my sister and I had to do about after care related to the surgery. There was a reasonable chance that my Mom might emerge from surgery partially paralyzed or substantially disabled, so those thoughts could not be pushed away; they had to be confronted directly.

The wait during the first surgery turned out, in retrospect, to have been probably the easiest part of the whole process because we were able to wait together as a family. We had also expected a much longer wait than what occurred. After only a few hours, a call came in to the desk nurse in the waiting area, and she called for someone from the family to come forward. Given how early it was in what was expected to be a six-plus-hour procedure, we had a fluttery moment—something could have gone wrong early in the procedure. However, the news was good and the doctors were very optimistic about how things had gone. I think we all started to think more concretely about the recovery stage.

Prior to the operation, my Mom had divided responsibility for her affairs between my sister and me. My sister was in charge of the financial end (which might have been of great significance had the procedure gone poorly), and I was in charge of the medical end. We were able to communicate well enough that there never was an issue on which we disagreed. As background, I was working in Oakland, California, as a high school teacher and coach when my Mom underwent the operation. I remember walking into the headmaster's office to let him know that I would need to resign my position, given the likely after-care needs associated with the procedure. Much to my amazement and gratitude, the school allowed me to take the time away from work; I would be able to commute to Oakland a couple of times a month for a few days to coach my team and join the team when they were competing on road trips.

During the time my Mom was in the hospital I tried to serve as

Carol R. Palo

her lead advocate. Never had my skills as a debate coach been put to a more effective use.

Mom left the hospital with a very positive prognosis and went first to a rehabilitation center and then home. My role was to continue to act as an advocate for her during recovery. When in Portland I lived in her home and, after she had returned home, did what I could to be a caregiver. Although her time in the hospital called upon the debate portion of my skills, her aftercare called upon the coach portion of that vocational background. Mom's meticulous adherence to her rehabilitation program made it a relatively easy role to play.

Being involved in such a process is bound to have some impact, and my situation was no exception. First, it brought my sister and me closer together. We had always gotten along very well, but one of the virtues of working together to address a crisis is that it tends to bond people. Working together to assist our mother had such an effect, I suspect, on both of us. Second, it gave me a chance to give back to my Mom, who had sacrificed a great deal in raising my sister and me, which was immensely rewarding. As I tried to encourage her to accept the help of others during her recovery, I consistently invoked this notion, which was clearly apparent in all those I observed who volunteered assistance during her recovery. Third, it helped me in discovering the limits of what I am capable of as well as how to manage myself as a resource in times of crisis. That skill has turned out to be of great use to me in subsequent endeavors.

My daughter, April

My mom had mentioned her back casually at about age 58, but we had not talked about it or taken it seriously. I don't remember exactly, but as it continued to progress and become more painful for her, she began to talk about alternatives like acupuncture. I don't think it was until she was 60 that I realized it was a health issue.

I believe I was concerned and very skeptical of acupuncture making an impact. It wasn't until we were outlet shopping and I went into her changing room for us to look at each other's outfits that it really hit me. I saw her without her shirt on and could see exactly how extreme the curve or bend was. I was very upset! It hit me really hard, and we finally had a real discussion about what was happening.

I definitely had fear that she would not make it through the surgery or that it would either make things worse or not improve them. The [second] surgery was so long and so extreme that it felt like there were too many things that could go amiss rather than go right. It really seemed like a long shot, but it was the only thing to do.

Waiting during surgery was very stressful. I don't remember much other than waiting by the phone and pacing. I think Oliver and Nick stayed home with me so that I wouldn't be by myself. We stuck together. The odd part of having it last for two days was that it seemed to keep going on and on. I remember when she got out of surgery and the doctor called because the second day of surgery went quicker than he thought it would. We drove to the hospital immediately. Because they hold a person after surgery for a bit before taking them to their room and because I had to drive so far, I got there just as she was being wheeled from the elevator to her room. The thing was, she was so bloated and puffy that I didn't recognize her at first, which also scared me. It's weird not to recognize your own mother and scary. I thought I was OK until then, and then I got scared again.

My brother and I took turns in the various roles of protector, advocate, worrier, child, etc. The great part was not being alone but having Nick and Oliver to be there for support so we could all feel what we needed to as we felt it. It was hard being "on" for my daughter, who was only about 18 months old. It's hard to put on a brave face when you are scared.

This situation definitely has changed me. I value life, health, family and my Mom much more than before. It is also amazing to see what you can live through and with. It is an experience that has made our family even stronger. I know that there is nothing that I wouldn't do for my family and I know that I can count on them for anything.

Carol R. Palo

My son-in-law, Oliver

I heard about the seriousness of the back problems from my wife after she first went with her mom to a doctor appointment. I felt uncertain, scared and solemn. I wondered if, after surgery, she would be able to live her life like she did before. During the surgery I was very anxious to see how it went. My support was mostly to help and assist my wife so that she could be free to help whenever needed. What I learned is to never take health issues as a joke.

Friends

Debi

- When Carol told me about her back problems and the surgery she would require I felt shocked and frightened. She is such a good friend and I could not believe it. Of course I thought of how I could help support or encourage her. It was really hard to believe that she had such a serious problem with her back because she had never even complained about it and I had known her for over fifteen years by this time.

- There was a point when Carol was icing her back just to get through work. One evening she called me and told me she had fallen and could not get back up, could I please come over and help her? I immediately drove over and was happy to have her greet me and open the door. As I recall she had recovered and was able to get up but her condition was becoming serious. It was at this time I knew she would need the surgery.

- The surgery process was a three day ordeal, one of the most intense I had ever experienced. I remember visiting Carol in the hospital the second day while she was in the "twilight" phase of the surgery. She had one side done and needed to rest before they worked on the other side. I remember going into the room and she was lying on her side as I recall "resting" to get prepared for the final surgery. I was gravely affected in ways I can't explain. Carol had told me she could come out of this with anything from a slight paralysis to even possible death. I felt very tense and worried for my dear friend. I tried to be supportive to her loving family and other friends.

- After the surgery, I tried to be part of the team to help with meals and other support as she recovered in rehab and at home. It was a long process for her.

- Having my close friend Carol go through this has changed me in many ways. First of all it makes me see more and more how important close friends are.

- I would just suggest be there for your friend or loved one going through this surgery. Try to be patient and listen to them. The entire process is so lengthy and overwhelming for the patient. I know my friend Carol is a very brave and courageous person. She wrote this book to help others who are having the same procedure.

Joe

Having known you for years, I knew you had back issues. A lot of that came from you sharing your travel stories and some of the issues you encountered in taking excursions. I don't remember when I heard about your surgery specifically.

I felt sorry; I felt it wasn't fair. I never felt any concern that the operation might not be successful. I just wanted to know how I could best help you.

I didn't visit you in the hospital as I understood that was not wanted. I visited you in the rehab center and later at home. From our talks at the rehab center we came up with a plan as to what you needed at home. I felt that we were friends and should the tables be turned, that you would be there for me.

I always had positive feelings about the surgery and my main focus came after surgery. I went to your new home and added some extra handrails and other features to help you move safely and comfortably through your home. For the first few months, Kate and I would come out on some Sundays and cook dinner, and arrange for people to come to visit and pray for your recovery.

Since I have also had numerous surgeries I am aware of the efforts that people went to in assisting you. It made me recognize and be even more appreciative of the help that I too received.

I recommend to any faced with such situations to do your research on doctors and hospitals; reach out and ask for help from your friends and neighbors. Most will be willing and able to help. It's not a time to isolate.

Clara

We met when you started work at the company where I was employed. I found out that you were having serious back problems and facing surgery a few years after meeting you. As the pain became worse you were more willing to reveal it saying that pain sometimes interfered with your sleep.

When you told me that your spine had curved as much as it could without harming your internal organs I was shocked and saddened. I was very impressed with research you conducted in order to choose the best surgeon for you. You interviewed doctors in California, Seattle and in Portland. I was happy that you chose the Portland doctor since that meant I would be near enough to assist you in any way I could.

I've never known anyone who has been through such an extreme surgery. I was so happy for you that your children were supportive and helped your friends by keeping us posted and also asking for what was needed from your friends. Prior to your surgery I held the vision that the surgery would go well and communicated to you that belief, which I think was reassuring to you. During the surgery your friends and I prayed for your complete recovery and continued holding the vision that your surgeon and surgical team would take excellent care of you. I also asked your angels to be with you and to work with the medical team's angels. After your move to the rehab facility I visited frequently, sometimes advocating for you when there was not a quick response from the staff. Those details escape me now. Once you were able to go home I visited there. A team of us cleaned house for you until you became well enough to do it yourself. We also planted flowers for your patio and in your yard. I was one of those friends who did whatever you needed that you couldn't do for yourself. Several of us provided some healing energy work as well as spiritual sustenance.

Accompanying you during your major (I call it extreme) surgery experience and the recovery process made it clear to me that we humans need each other. With enough money you could have purchased all the services that your friends and family provided. Purchased services aren't always provided with love and caring as you found out with the home health nurse you wanted to ban from caring for you. So yes, accompanying you through your surgery and recovery changed me. I hope that I am now less fiercely independent and more able to accept help if and when I need it. It was such a joy working with the rest of your friends to help you recover full independence. And I've gained a deeper appreciation for shared spiritual sustenance.

My advice to anyone facing major surgery is to choose their healthcare team and facilities wisely and to keep your family and friends informed as to your progress and needs. People want to help and just need to know what would be helpful. I think the whole process requires as much as any other major event. It helps to have someone know and broadcast the timeline, locations, and who is going to do what and when. It also helped that you were so thoughtful and grateful for everything that anyone did for you. When we came to your house to clean or just visit you had food you thought we would like, you asked about us and our lives. You were good at answering questions about your process but also careful to see that our helping you wasn't just about you. Your surgery was a success in many ways. You are now taller and not slanted to one side. You learned the depth of your friendships. You learned that you are loved and not alone.

Wow, what an experience! So glad it's over and hoping that those of us who shared this experience with you continue to feel the flow of connection.

Steff

1. I knew Carol was having back trouble soon after I met her at work. She shared more about the degenerative effects of her scoliosis and we talked at length about what kinds of decisions may have to be made and how she evaluated some of the options. Then after a few years, Carol actually had to face the choices and make a decision before things became irreversible.

2. I instantly thought Carol would make the right decision for her. Carol taught me along the way that you have to make decisions you are willing to live with and to be accountable for. I hoped that she would decide on surgery. It was the only option she could make that would allow her to live the life she so diligently built for herself.

3. I always knew that not only myself, but all of her friends and family would support her, and I knew that she would tell us what she needed from us, and when and how to do it for her. . . she would do the same for any of us (she would make us let her help).

4. When I saw her as the Goodyear tire man in the intensive care unit. . .I knew she would have a long road and I saw how brave she was. I immediately thought that should anything like this come up for me or my family, that we should do it sooner rather than later, and that we should make sure we cover all of our bases the way Carol did.

5. I think I helped Carol more spiritually than physically. Our trip to Seattle to meet with her (then) potential doctor was full of her detailed research, yet fun as usual as she looked at this as a project and made the best of our long day.

6. I made the comment to my husband that Carol taught me two things during this time and throughout our friendship
   1) You have to be the best you can be.
   2) You have friends for a reason and you're a good friend for a reason.

7. If you need to do anything for yourself either medically or drastically life-changing (even for a short period of time), be thorough and line up your support system early. Carol remained independent and successful because she covered her bases, and made things as comfortable for herself and others as possible. A positive attitude was Carol's legacy during this time, and I think throughout her life.

Carol R. Palo

We must be willing to get rid of the life we planned,
so as to have the life that is waiting for us.
—Joseph Campbell

CHAPTER 8

OTHER JOURNEYS

~⌒

A few special friends and acquaintances agreed to share their unexpected medical situations as well. Each of us had to draw on resources, face fears, financial or insurance situations, and resources both material and spiritual to create a broader look at how we deal with life's unknowns. My thanks go to all those who made such a difference for me.

Joe and the motorcycle accident

I remember exactly—Aug. 23, 1976. As a drunk driver approached hitting me head on while I was on my motorcycle, time slowed way down. I thought about how I might avoid getting hit and then saw there was no way to avoid it. I moved to the center of my lane, slowing down…maybe it was at the point of contact, but there was a moment when I was surrounded by a white light and knew that no matter what happened, I'd be alright.

The ambulance drivers apologized for arriving so late. When they got the call with details of what had happened, they just assumed I was dead. In fact the hospital placed me in a room by the morgue, assuming I was not going to make it. On my left side, I had a dislocated hip, broken leg and broken foot. My right side was pretty banged up too. Fortunately, I was wearing a motorcycle helmet. It split open and my head was swelling up. There were fears of brain damage. This was the beginning of a long journey.

1 1/2 years of not being able to work followed as a result of the accident. Since I had no income my family and I moved in with my parents. They gave me the 2nd floor of their house and took care of everything. I couldn't even get down the stairs for six months. The hardest thing was asking anyone for help and accepting it.

Over the years I have gone through six knee surgeries and a hip replacement.

As the shock of the accident wore off, I felt like everything— my progress, life, relationships were unfolding. I don't know if the unfolding ever really stops but at some point a new way of living life takes over and the sense of living in trauma fades away. But the accident and its aftermath changed me and the directions of my life. The difficulties weren't helpful in the marriage and played a part in its disintegration ending in divorce. However, because of the time I spent at my parents' home getting to know my children very well, I was awarded sole custody of them, 8 and 10 years old at the time. This wouldn't have happened had I not spent this special time with them. I had a great attorney who was successful in ensuring that my health insurance company covered all the hospital bills. The settlement from the auto insurance was kept separate so that I had funds to be able to cover some of the future surgeries. Horror stories about insurance companies are common, but my health insurance stepped in and picked up bills while who was paying what was being decided.

My life was all about change. Some I accepted and some I couldn't. My energies went into every way that I could remove the physical limitations placed on me by the doctors. I couldn't get past all of them, but I surprised a lot of people with what I could do. The down side of such determination was that I eventually needed to slow down and act more responsibly toward my body.

The question is: where am I today as someone who has survived a catastrophic event? Physically, I live as normally as possible but have needed surgeries on knees and hips over the years in order to keep moving. In terms of my thinking, emotions and spirituality, I have learned to move through each day just as it happens. I still have strong emotions when thinking about the accident and when discussing it (which isn't often). I feel blessed to be where I am in my life today and it has caused me to value and become closer to family members. I am able to understand why my dad always stressed how important it was to keep the family whole.

For anyone who is going through a difficult medical situation or is a family member or friend I can offer the following. The brain is more powerful than we know. Keep things as positive as possible and don't doom patients with information or predictions that might not be true. It really helps to remember there are always options and it's the small steps that lead to success.

Patti and lung cancer

A cough and a cold just wouldn't go away. So off to the doctor, he prescribed antibiotics and insisted I get a lung X-ray. The X-ray showed I had pneumonia. After taking the antibiotics and feeling better, the doctor wanted me to get a follow-up X-ray. This was something I normally wouldn't have wanted to deal with but I got the X-ray anyhow. My doctor called and said, "It doesn't look good. You have a tumor in one lung and we need to do a biopsy." The biopsy confirmed it was stage four, small cell cancer, very dangerous. Next I was sent to an oncologist to talk about surgery and treatment. The news was startling, but the doctor seemed to be very competent and reassuring. The oncologist felt the safest way to rid me of cancer was to take out the left lobe of my lung where it was located, biopsy the lymph nodes during surgery to be sure they had all of it and then treatments of chemotherapy to get anything that may be hiding throughout the body. I was sent to see a lung surgeon. I had a lot of questions, little by little they were answered, but I had to have family remind me and also write things down. I just wanted to get it done, but first I had to take several tests. I was a long time smoker so they needed to do heart and breathing strength tests. This took another few weeks; about a month had gone by since the X-ray and I was on leave from work, blessed I had insurance. Finally, I went into surgery, feeling scared but accepted this was the thing to do. The option was very grim and unspeakable. It seemed easiest to just not deal with any feelings at that time and simply put one foot in front of the other. After surgery, as I lay in my hospital bed, I couldn't believe the amount of pain I was in. The nurses gave me all the medication allowable but it didn't seem to help much. I also had an allergic reaction to some of the medication that added to my misery. They got me on my feet and moving as soon as possible. I know they were so insistent because it is critical to recovery, but it was really rough. After eight days I was using a walker. Friends and family came to visit often. Although they were very encouraging, I was too miserable most of the time to care. Going home was hard.

Even harder were the oncologist's words that came a few weeks later. He said I would need extensive chemotherapy. Maybe the scariest part of that was being told I shouldn't work during this time if I wanted to get the greatest benefits from the chemo. My sixty days of short term disability would be ending, and there would be a four month time gap before any long term disability funds would be available. My employer kept me on the books so I had continued insurance but no money to live on. Thank goodness for a relative who loaned me the money for that interim time. It was hard to accept this help but I had to adjust my attitude. SSDI was applied for and denied. It would take lawyers two years and three denials before they took over for the long term disability. I received less money but had insurance.

There were positives that came from the ordeal. I found out how truly supportive my friends and family were even when they were clearly disappointed at my continued struggles to stop smoking. My daughter and I became closer. I strengthened my sense of spirituality and saw how much it helped during the cancer treatments and how much it could help with all things. I was able to help a friend go through breast cancer with more awareness and empathy.

Today, when challenged, I can say to myself, "I got through cancer with the help of others and there's not much else to be afraid of." Recommitting to my spirituality has been really good for my belief system. I've had to look at my vanity and ego, vulnerability and the permanent physical changes that have come. I am clearer on what is really important as a person, and have developed more patience and tolerance. I've become more able to accept life on life's terms.

For anyone reading my story I can offer the following:

If you have a serious medical situation, please remember to fight and keep your balance in your heart and head. Be very firm until all your questions are answered. Remember it is your life [and] maybe you will choose an unpopular option, if so be sure to speak to medical people and a spiritual adviser before the family. Doctors, nurses and support people to help with money, living, food, clothing etc. each have their part in your situation. They are not really indifferent but just have specific areas of expertise that they will discuss with you. This keeps them honest and not speculating; in the long run this is less confusing and frightening. Do not get ahead of their process; they need all the facts first.

For family and friends I can offer how important it is to show how hopeful you are and please do not personalize the affront against yourself. In so many situations, a little lightness and humor is welcome and much needed.

Regarding the medical people, I can say that my experience made me thankful for their expertise and honest attitudes. I was grateful that my doctors made sure they had a second opinion from others in their practice. To all I came across during my sickness and healing I always knew they wanted to help me and do all in their power to make me well again.

Ed and unexpected open-heart surgery

I've always been physically active. Then I noticed that when running or even walking I would get really tired. I was taking blood pressure medication and assumed it to be the cause. That summer, I couldn't mow the lawn without stopping half way through to rest. I finally went to the doctor, explaining I felt lethargic and asking to have the medication dose checked. My doctor wanted me to take a stress treadmill test that Tues. and I complied. The tester just walked away and told me he couldn't analyze the results. I was told the test just didn't go well. When I talked to my cardiologist she said I needed an angiogram—the next day! I couldn't see the need for such a rush and had no idea that this was a serious procedure. But I did show up and even thought to ask my wife if she wanted to be there. During the angiogram they said they saw blockage everywhere and need to perform open-heart surgery immediately. I wanted to slow the whole situation down to get a second opinion and look at my options but they said the situation was serious enough that there was no time for second opinions or anything else. They planned to keep me in the hospital and perform the surgery the next day.

The reality is that life wasn't the same as way back before surgery when I had no real health issues. During convalescence, I became very depressed and felt I had become less of a person than before. I didn't feel whole physically. I felt flawed and of less value. I didn't see how being home alone was very isolating and probably contributing to the depression. Fortunately my wife noticed. This led to serious conversations and made me aware that the relationship with my wife had become deeper and more meaningful to me. A time came when I literally felt angels dancing on my chest. This wasn't emotional but truly a physical experience. After that, I felt whole again and the depression lifted.

Today, many years later, I still work out every day and can acknowledge that I am less able physically than earlier in my life. There doesn't seem to be any long term effect on my family as a result of the surgery or convalescence period. I have a sensitivity to the cold I never had before, but that is most likely a combination of being older and the lack of enough coronary arteries. I have gained awareness that life is a gift. I have experienced anger at God for a genetic predisposition to heart problems because it affects my emotional state and keeps me from doing all that I want to do

Marilyn's scoliosis

I was fourteen. My mom was on a chaise lounge by the side of the pool at the deep end. After I accomplished a quick dive off the side, she commanded that I come over next to her. She told me to stand up straight! I stood up straight and she ordered again, "No, stand up straight!"

"I am standing up straight!" I yelled back.

"Well, you're crooked. We're going to take you to the doctor."

And so the journey began.

I was feeling rather sorry for myself and didn't want to tell anyone. After all I was almost fifteen and really boy crazy. Who'd want to date someone who is deformed? My mother was concerned if she would ever be a grandmother. Would anyone want to marry her deformed daughter? I think she was more upset than I was. Fortunately, my dad was, as always, in my court for support and encouragement.

It took a long time to develop X-rays in 1964. Finally the doctors confirmed the already known diagnosis. The doctor laid my X-rays on a table that had a light source underneath. He got out a measuring tape and measured my spine on the X-ray from the top to the bottom. Then he got out a long string and laid the string along the backwards S-curve of the spine at the same starting and ending spot and made another measurement. The difference was four inches. If my spine had been straight, instead of being 5'2" I would have been 5'6"!

The doctor said there were two choices. I could have physical therapy or surgery. He explained that if I opted for the surgery, I'd have a single Harrington rod attached to my spine and be in a cast for several months. Then I would wear a brace for at least six months. They'd have to do the surgery right away before my epiphyseal plates sealed. This meant before I stopped growing anymore, because if I waited the bones would be set and it couldn't be corrected. In addition, my spine would have to be fused. That would significantly hamper my mobility. Physical therapy was sounding really good by now! He suggested I also hang two parallel, horizontal rods in a doorway and hang from them for at least ten minutes a day. He said I should hang with my left hand on the top rod and the right hand on the bottom rod. He advised that if I stayed active the rest of my life, I shouldn't have too many problems and should be able to have children. Since I was athletic and good at sports, it was clear that my course of action would be physical therapy.

So I was a normal, but slightly deformed teenager. From the front you would never have noticed. The curve was only apparent when I bent over and was viewed from the back. Except for gym class, it was easy to look like everyone else. I dated, played sports, and told no one about my spine. The peer pressure to be "perfect" is pretty intense for teenage girls. Life went on. I attended college, had some great jobs, got married and had a child.

When I was in my mid to late thirties, I worked for a high tech company and I visited lots of customers. At one customer site I met with a woman to help her with software. When I bent over to show her something on her screen she exclaimed "Oh, you have scoliosis!" I hated it when people occasionally pointed it out to me. Those reminders would always leave me feeling badly for many days afterwards. But she got my attention when she added "I had a surgery to correct that a year and a half ago. I'm doing great. It was the best thing I could have done!" I asked for her doctor's name and immediately knew someday I would have it done too.

I interviewed two doctors and decided on the one my customer had referred me to. Then came the dreaded X-rays and curve measuring. During pregnancy, my bones softened and it really did a number on the scoliosis. I had noticed, when trying on bathing suits, the curve had gotten worse. He measured the curves and the upper curve was 59 degrees and the lower curve was 42 degrees. He told me that when the top curve got to 60 degrees, my spine would start impairing my lung function. Yikes! I was turning forty and it was time for surgery.

I prepared for the surgery for almost a year. I was a workout maniac. I also used lots of positive message tapes that were mostly soothing music with subliminal messages. I did a lot of research. My son was five at the time and I tried to prepare him for a time when mommy would be away for a while and need lots of attention from him and his daddy. I even considered making a tape for him of me in case I wouldn't be there anymore. I also had concerns about something going wrong and being left paralyzed or less than lucid. I was very scared.

The surgery went well and I was stable enough to go to a regular hospital room. Yea – I didn't die on the operating table!

The doctors wanted me to get up and walk on day three. The pain had lessened but I didn't think I could get up. My 5 year old son visited for the first time. I was worried he would be upset to see me in the hospital. I forgot how resilient kids are. He was fine and just happy to see me. By day 5 the doctors insisted I get up, eat solid food and dine in a chair rather than in bed. I felt like I might pass out, but did everything they asked. By the next day I was walking around the hospital feeling very much like myself again. Not only that, but when they measured me I had grown almost two inches!

I was in the hospital for one week. My incision was closed with surgical staples—lots of them. I couldn't take a shower or wash my hair, or even bend over the sink until the staples came out. The staples were removed after about another week and it felt good to get really clean.

I was glad to leave the hospital, but scared, because I felt so fragile. I felt like I might break and was afraid to do anything but be upright, walk around or lay down. One of the first things I did after getting home was look at myself in a full length mirror. It was amazing. I was tall and straight and smiling. Yes, I had staples in my back and greasy hair but I was straight!

Here is some recovery advice for spinal surgery patients:

- Don't sneeze. I didn't sneeze for almost a year. I actually sneezed once and it hurt so badly that I vowed to not do that again.
- Avoid friends who always greet you with bear hugs. Some people just can't help themselves, even when reminded about the back surgery.
- The metal rods actually feel cold in the winter, if you live in a cold climate, at least for the first couple of years.
- At first, sleeping is elusive. Your normal sleep positions probably aren't possible.
- Let people help you! Because muscles were cut during surgery, I also was unable to lift anything. I couldn't even get milk out of the refrigerator. This left my son feeling very manly as the strong person of the house during the day. It was good for me and great for him.
- For me the short term recovery was very short. I thought I'd be lying in bed for weeks, but aside from napping, I was never in bed except at night.
- The longer term recovery can take a year or two and is greatly aided by exercise. I did warm water aerobics as soon as my doctor allowed. Walking (flat areas are better) helped build up strength and stamina as well.
- Make things easy on yourself. Really use the tools available to help get things done and be more independent.
- You may have strange physical feelings like tingling as the nerves try to hook back up to each other. You might also have areas that are numb. Some of these feel normal after a while and some

of them don't, but it all takes a long time. Even today, twenty three years later, I still get the "tinglies" across the back of my shoulders when I am really tired.

The not so great stuff:

Sometimes there are side effects doctors won't attribute to the surgery, but they are problems you never had prior to surgery. In my case it was vertigo. About three months after the surgery, I was turning over in bed and suddenly the room started spinning around. After visits to many doctors (Western and Chinese medicine), acupuncturists, and physical therapists, I have just learned to live with it. I don't have it all the time, but when I do, it is very annoying. Also, at first, I was worried I had a brain tumor or something really serious. I didn't need that extra stress.

The most important thing is, I live a normal life with an (almost) straight spine and have been able to enjoy my family and work.

PART THREE
HELPFUL TOOLS AND
RESOURCES

We can't control our destiny, but we can control who we become.
—Anne Frank

CHAPTER 9

QUESTIONNAIRES, CHARTS, AND IDEAS

*F*or me, unwanted change translates into a sense of chaos. I think it's probably the same feeling for most people. A format for organizing and expressing questions, worries, goals, and random thoughts helped me achieve at least a small sense of empowerment and direction.

Part III contains lists, questions, ideas, and some examples of my entries, with space for you to add and create your own. If something doesn't make sense or apply to you, leave it out and add what will help you. I also include more detailed information on actions I took and ideas I used. We can find our own personal balance of practical information and emotional relief with activities that minimize the difficult times.

I hope these ideas are helpful in finding the right path for you.

The First Week: Coming-to-Terms-with List: A Questionnaire and Thoughts

WHAT ARE POSITIVE THOUGHTS ABOUT MY SITUATION?

- I have time to decide about whether to have surgery or not.
- Other doctors might have more options.
- I have available a really good support base of family and friends if I ask them for help.
-
-
-

WHAT ARE MY FEARS?

- Will I be crippled and end up in chronic pain before I'm even ready to retire?
- Will I lose my job?
- Will my insurance cover whatever I need to have done medically and if not, how will I pay for it?
-
-
-

WHAT POSITIVE RESOURCES DO I HAVE?

- Years ago a friend had a similar problem in her upper back. She had successful surgery and would understand what I am going through.
- I have a friend who survived cancer and changed her entire lifestyle. She is a survivor with the courage to do whatever it takes to have quality of life.
- I have an adult son and daughter who will stand by me and help me no matter what.
-
-
-

Here are good ideas from a few friends, my son, and daughter (the few people I called in the first 24 hours after the doctor visit).

- Get references from people who had the surgery.
- Go to a back specialty shop and check out equipment like a zero gravity chair.
- Call friends I trust for reality checks.
- Remember that whatever happens—surgery, debilitation—I'm still me and will still be loved.
- Try to separate out my fears and emotional distress from what is really happening to my body.

WHAT DO I WANT TO DO BEFORE I AM EITHER BADLY CRIPPLED OR HAVE SURGERY?

- I want to take my family to see the Blue Man Group show in Las Vegas.
- I want to travel as much as possible.
- I want to be active and pay attention to how much I enjoy it while I still can.
-
-
-

WHAT IS MY TO-DO LIST PRIOR TO SURGERY OR BEING TOO DISABLED TO WORK?

- Check insurance and disability plan.
- Do my best work to be as sure as possible to keep my job.
- Make out a real will and a directives form.
- Start a list of concerns I have about activities I can now do that might be affected:
    - Driving a car
    - Having sex
    - Walking up and down stairs
    - Pain management
    -

Thoughts of Gratitude

These are grateful thoughts and a sense of direction that came to me while sitting in a beautiful garden (surprisingly enough, I could still feel gratitude or appreciation even though I was afraid and angry). Please add what you feel gratitude for and what makes you feel hopeful.

THANK YOU GOD

- For all this beauty.
- For enough grace to turn this corner and be able to get up and get on with my life.
- For right now, at least, feeling that the fear has moved to an outer ring on the bull's eye of my new horizon.
- For knowing I can still think and plan and have a good day today.
-
-
-

Random thoughts from the first week after the first doctor visit

- The last couple of days I've felt like I'm coming down with the flu or a cold, or maybe it's just a stress reaction to what's going on.
- Surgery concerns: Am I too old to handle up to twenty hours of anesthetic? What if it affects my mind permanently? I haven't even told the doctor yet about my other health issues.
-
-
-
-

Questions to ask each doctor

I thought that a list of questions I would ask each doctor made sense, just like going out for bids on a business proposal. If everyone is asked the same questions, it's easier to compare what is being offered. My list is a combination of what the first doctor suggested (yes, I asked him what he would ask if it was his back) and questions that just came to me.

1. What is your prognosis, both the severity of my problems and options that would be surgical and nonsurgical?
2. Why do you make that prognosis and indicate those options?
3. What will you do to determine the exact nature of my spinal problems?
4. Do you have a team you generally work with on these types of surgeries?
5. How many similar surgeries have you performed, and what are the success stats in detail?
6. I will be getting other opinions. Is there someone else you would recommend my seeing?
7. What do you recommend I do next?
8. Can I keep or get a copy of X-rays or tests you order?
9. What do you see as a realistic scenario if I don't have surgery?
10. At this point will pushing myself with physical activity be of any structural value or will it hurt me?
11.
12.
13.
14.
15.
16.
17.
18.

Making sense of information from doctors and other medical professionals

You can read through all your notes or create a chart with your questions. Decide which is easier for you. If you use a chart, try to fill it in after each healthcare provider meeting. Assigning a number to each question gives you the flexibility to use either the number or the question in future notes or charts.

Don't get too carried away with getting every question answered or not feeling you can ask other questions. The point of the chart is to help you keep track of what is being presented to you so you can make the most informed decisions about what you will do next.

For example:

	Dr A	Dr B	Physical therapist
1. Q: What treatment?	wear brace,exercise	surgery	learn techniques
2. Q: Why surgery?	too risky	best option	deal with losing mobility
3. Q: Details of plan			
4. Q:			
5. Q:			
6. Q:			

Comments or observations after medical visits
- All doctors agree surgery is risky.
- Look at resolving pain or more permanent solution.
- Check again best ways suggested to deal with plain.

Tips for Selecting Health Care Providers

- Document every conversation and save any material you receive. Even notes to yourself with names, dates, and basic info will become handy.
- If you don't have insurance, check the Internet, old-fashioned phone books for local agencies that might have information or assistance, and tips from friends. As of 2012, there is a huge difference in availability from state to state. Take a chance on asking for assistance; hearing "No we can't help you" several times is worth it for the one "Yes, here's what's available to you." Be very careful if any of these sources wants to charge you to help you get information. There are a lot of scam artists and organizations that prey on people needing assistance.
- If you have insurance, contact your carrier and find out exactly what coverage you have, how to get the bills paid, what choices you have in selecting the doctors and procedure, getting second opinions, and costs to you for any outside-the-network care.
- If surgery is being considered, get at least a second opinion, preferably from a doctor connected to a different clinic.
- If surgery or other procedure or care suggested carries risks, prior to making a decision ask for references so you can contact patients who have already gone through it. Finding out how other patients feel about the experience or knowing that the doctor won't give you references can be critical to making a good decision.

I don't want to be treated like I'm just a number or body part

Many medical providers who deal with taking X-rays, setting up MRIs, examining data and injury pain sites, or taking down information all day need to place some emotional distance between themselves and the difficult stories each circumstance represents. So it is easy for those of us who are patients to feel we are being treated like just a body part or a number. It can be empowering if we choose to show a little compassion for those assisting us in tracking down what's happening to our bodies. Here are also a few things we can do to remind others that we are still valid and present.

- If people are talking about you as if you aren't really there, joke around a little. You can say something like, "By the way, I'm connected to that elbow (or spine) and I have questions," or "I'm in pain," or "I can answer that for you."
- When friends or family members repeatedly ask how the elbow or spine is, answer them but also add comments like, "And the rest of me is pretty good today, too" or "Actually, the spine is only part of the pain because the rest of me is uncomfortable, too," or, "The whole rest of me is still attached to the elbow. I'm taking care of business but anxious about what comes next."
- Introduce yourself and ask for the names of the people assisting you. If it seems appropriate, call them by name, offer a little information about yourself, and ask how their day is going. Creating a little friendly conversation, if time allows, helps both you and the provider to connect in a more human and personal way.
- If you have surgery and will be unable to communicate for more than a day, make up a little poster and hang it in your room. It will show your care providers who you are as a person with information like, "My name is Carol and I will be visited here by my son, daughter and friends. I need to take _____ medications each morning. Here is a photo of me without all the tubes and looking happy. I love dogs and share a Sheltie with my granddaughter. I own an overly sensitive bamboo plant."
- Add any scenarios of your own.

Chart used both before and after surgery to track "How am I doing?"

Across the top of the page, space out numbers from 0 to 10. Down the left side of the page enter two columns. One indicates what you are measuring; the other indicates the date or time. This chart can help you keep track of what you are really feeling in terms of pain, stress, or whatever you are measuring. Just put an *x* or check mark under the number that applies: 0 indicates no pain or problem and 10 indicates lots as in too much. Sometimes seeing the actual numbers is healthier than rationalizing or ignoring what is going on inside. Don't get caught up in measuring as a new hobby, however. Taking stock in the morning and again in the afternoon or evening is probably enough. See the example below and modify to suit your needs.

		0	1	2	3	4	5	6	7	8	9	10
Pain-spine	9/13 2pm											x
Pain-spine	9/13 10pm											x
Sleepless-fear	9/14 2am											x
Pain-spine	9/14 5am							x				
Pain walking	9/14 11am		x									
Sleepless-fear	9/17 1am							x				

Final version: To-Do List prior to surgery

This list continues your first To-Do List prior to surgery or major disability. Anything not yet completed on that list is a good start for the new list. If you have a surgery date scheduled, you'll need a space for each item that needs to be done and by which date prior to the surgery date. The example below is similar to what I used prior to surgery. I wanted all items completed one week prior, so I entered a due by date only when it needed to be done earlier. Please add to it or adjust it to fit your needs and responsibilities.

- Have newspaper stopped for the estimated time of surgery and rehabilitation.
- Arrange for family member to pick up my mail and sort through, throwing out all but bills and important documents or correspondence. The post office will hold mail up to 30 days if that turns out to work better.
- Talk to boss and HR about when I need to leave and why. Discuss who will do my job and what is involved. DO BY JUNE 1st.
- Tell coworkers about being out of the office and who is doing my job or work while I am gone and when I expect to be back. I want to be careful that I give accurate information about why I will be out of the office, but not so much that I feel uncomfortable or so much that I make other people uncomfortable. DO BY AUG 10th.
- Read all information from the hospital and doctor to be sure I am ready for check-in.
- Let friends know about upcoming surgery and that I will need help afterward. Write down names of everyone who says they would be willing to help at all. DO BY AUG 10th.

Questions to ask doctor regarding post-surgery to be asked at least 30 days prior to surgery

The answers to these questions and any you add or substitute will help you and those assisting you figure out what to do to help ensure a smooth and quick recovery.

- Will I be able to use stairs, and how long after a successful surgery would that be (my house has stairs with my bedroom upstairs)?
- Will I be able to do basic skills like put on my socks, wipe myself in the bathroom, and take a shower? What about moving my arms overhead to dress myself?
- After surgery, how long will I be in the brace and what kind of brace is it?
- Since I live alone, will I be self-sufficient enough to go home directly from the hospital?
- After I leave the hospital, what kind of care will I need to heal and return to normal activities?
- If a family member or friend comes by every day, will that be enough help?
- Will I need physical therapy or anything else to become as functional as possible?

Methods of relieving stress prior to surgery: physical, mental, emotional

Stress of any type takes up huge amounts of energy. Add that to the amount of stress consumed dealing with pain, and not much is left to deal with everyday living or new decisions that need to be made. Listed below are suggestions, in no particular order, to relieve stress. I've gone into detail on some of them because they were so helpful to me. I want you to know the process, so consider these and try some to discover which work best for you.

Physical movement depends on the degree of pain you are living with. The most important factor is tension relief, both mental and physical, that comes from getting enough blood flowing through the body and aids the muscles in staying functional.

- If physical therapists are available to you, try a few visits to see if they can assist you in developing some exercises that help you maintain or adjust your normal activities as long as possible. By the time I decided to try physical therapy, the visits were only depressing and painful because I had already passed the point when I could do any of the work suggested.
- Exercise classes or videos can help in staying mobile and, with music or other people involved, can be fun. It's important to remember you may need to check your ego at the door; you may have to massively adapt the exercises to fit your abilities.
- If you are currently involved in any sports, stay involved as long as your doctor and your pain level allow, even if your ability to perform well lessens.
- Walking, swinging your arms, stretching, movement in general every day can be done without cost, special gear, or instruction. Don't wait until the mood strikes you; just do what you can each day.
- Your daily routine can become increasingly difficult. If so, make a list of what you need to do each day starting with the most

important. I needed to get to work, get home, eat dinner quickly, and go upstairs to my bedroom or I would be in too much pain to eat or navigate the stairs. Having a priority plan allowed me do the basic activities more often.

- Add your own ideas.

Mental and emotional states can be rationalized or ignored, but they generally play out in some unpleasant, unexpected ways if not dealt with. The pressures of an uncertain future, fear, pain, and anger created distance between me and my friends. I'm not by nature someone who isolates; I just didn't want to communicate, think, or do anything. The following activities were my saving grace, allowing me to live as fully as possible in my circumstances. I still use these tools today.

- Laughter uses and relaxes muscles. It takes the edge off and activates those parts of the brain that tell us we feel better. This is not just my experience, but is verified in scientific experiments. Watch funny shows on your computer or TV, get together with people who are happy and like to laugh, read a funny book. Start collecting humorous quotes and jokes. Read them and share them as often as possible. Add your own ideas.
- Nature—just being outside with fresh air, sand, water, earth—has a way of calming and simplifying our insides (not, of course, during violent weather!). I could take a walk or sit in an area with plants and open sky, although it doesn't work well along with multitasking or even talking or texting on the phone. The trick is simply to focus on nature, noting what scents are there, seeing the clouds, really seeing each flower or tree branch. I was always amazed how just ten or fifteen minutes could help me to relax and feel more upbeat.
- Visualization, to me, is a means of stepping away from the moment's stresses, moving to a relaxing place, and returning rejuvenated without needing to move physically. No mind-altering

drugs or special training are needed. I hope anyone reading this will keep an open mind and try at least one of the suggested visualizations below. There is nothing to lose but a few minutes of your time. The benefit could be finding a simple way to have a more productive and healthy day.

- Example #1—on the beach: sit comfortably or stand in a relaxed manner and close your eyes. You could substitute a trip to the mountains if you prefer, but I like to use the beach. Breathe in and out slowly a few times and note that you can now feel warm, crunchy sand between your toes. The sun is warm and there is a slight breeze. Continue to breathe in and out slowly, and let yourself feel the sensations of sand, sun, and breeze. With your eyes still closed, imagine glimpsing a kite flying. Note the colors of the kite and see the clouds. Note if the clouds are puffy or look like ships, faces, or whatever else you can imagine. Breathe in and out slowly, and notice the sound of the ocean. The regular sound of waves rolling into the shore is almost hypnotic. Take a few minutes to focus on the sound of the ocean, the feeling of the sun and sand. Breathe in and out. Slowly open your eyes and notice how relaxed you feel.

- Example #2—the stairs: Sit or stand comfortably and close your eyes. Breathe in and out slowly and be open to visualize a tall stairway. It can be straight or curved, with or without a handrail. When you see your stairs, move toward them and start slowly climbing upward. At each step think of something that is bothering you, weighing you down. It can be physical pain, fear, or disappointment. At each step name one of these and drop it to the floor below. Proceed to the top of the stairs. The stairway can have any number of steps between five and ten. At the top of the stairs, stop and breathe in and out a few times. Think about feeling lighter than you were at the bottom of the stairs. If you wish, open the door at the top of the stairs and enter a garden. You can just stand there and enjoy the view, or go into the garden and enjoy the plants, water features, and whatever else is in your garden before opening your eyes and returning to your day.

- Example #3— This personal visualization came to me after many afternoons sitting in my actual backyard watching the birds and plants, waiting for an answer to how I could deal with my fears and future. I used this often prior to surgery, after surgery, and still do today. I'm relating it here as I visualize it:

    I'm sitting at the back of a small boat, like a canoe. It is rustic, not painted. The seat is a wooden board, and I have my hands in my lap. There is no need to move them or do anything but sit in the boat. We are on the water, which is without any ripples or movement. Tall reeds surround the boat. The air is so still that one could hear the sounds of a fly's wings moving. There is nothing but still-ness, gray-green water, and gray-green sky. I see at the front of the boat a figure in a dark cloak that also covers its head. The figure has its back to me, and it has a long pole in its hand. The pole is used to move the boat forward, and we glide silently, farther away from the shore. I somehow know that this is not a round-trip ride. We might make shore very close by or far away. But wherever we land, I will get out of the boat and go on with my life. For now, there is nothing to do but sit in the boat and peacefully go forward.

- Spirituality and religion are sometimes separate experiences. Whatever you believe, even if it is neither, do what you can to draw strength and guidance from your belief system. If like-minded people are available, they can be very helpful, too.
- Using interesting things to focus on and think about outside my medical situation were critical to me in finding the balance

between paying attention to what I needed to do for my health and morbid reflection on what was happening to me. Whether it was focusing on my job, gardening, helping other people, or watching a movie, just getting outside of my own mind and problems for a while relaxed me and gave me perspective. As my limitations became greater, it also helped me to still feel valuable and able to contribute. Make a list of what you do and could do if you find yourself locked in your problems.

- Gratitude vs. self-pity is a saving grace but hard to latch on to and maintain. I found it so helpful to keep the ability of seeing the good still happening in my life. Getting caught up in the unfairness of my situation, fears, anger at lack of choices I wanted, would lead to a sort of paralysis. I couldn't seem to think straight or care about much. I would isolate from the people who cared about me and could have offered hope and love. So for me, making sure to stay more in gratitude and less in self-pity was a strong way I could put quality into my daily life. I suggest you make a point of thinking about at least three things you are or could be grateful for every day.

Carol R. Palo

Finances and insurance list

It may be human nature to avoid subjects that are unpleasant to deal with, but it became a dubious luxury for me when it came to my finances and insurance issues. I knew it would be many months before I would be able to handle my finances on my own or keep track of insurance company requests for information. I also needed to know what my insurance would cover regarding the care I would need after leaving the hospital. I suggest the following as a guideline:

- Talk to your doctor about whether you can go directly home, what kind of specific care you will need, and for how long.
- If your doctor says you should get interim care rather than go directly home, contact your insurance company and find out what it covers and what paperwork is needed for approval.
- Your normal monthly or quarterly bills will need attention. If you are fortunate enough to have the assets, pay your monthly bills ahead of time. Paying online when possible is probably the easiest way. If you share finance issues with others in your household, make sure they know what you usually do, where the paperwork is, and how you do it.
- Be sure you have the appropriate contacts at your insurance company and know how to reach them in the most direct way. If precertifications are needed, find out when and what you are expected to do to make sure these are in place.
- Get a manual folder or binder to keep all the medically related paperwork in one place. Use tabs or pockets to separate information, material you need to complete and send somewhere, invoices, and anything else that's related. Creating a spreadsheet online to track payments, services, and medical supplies and prescriptions is the easiest way not to lose your mind while tracking the details.

What Comes Next, Including Post-Surgery Questions

Am I ready for the next phase of recovery and living? I think this is the guiding question after surgery. It applies as well to moving forward even if the decision is made not to have surgery. Whether preparing to leave the hospital or just making the current living situation more practical, some thoughts about what needs to change and how to make the changes must occur. Without preparation the results can involve more pain, additional loss of the ability to function, and lower quality of life than might be necessary. Please use the questions that apply to your own situation and ignore the rest. I hope that in answering the questions you will come up with others of your own.

- Based on what my physician says, how long do I have before I need to leave the hospital?
- Does the doctor know about my current living situation, and what does the doctor recommend in terms of aftercare?
- What kind of aftercare do I need?
    - Does it require skilled care, or can a family member or friend provide the care needed?
    - How long will I need that level of care?
    - If skilled care is needed, in what format or location does the doctor recommend?
    - If special care is needed, will anyone at the hospital help coordinate between the care provider or facility, my insurance, and the hospital?
    - If the answer to the last question is no, who could assist me in this coordination?
    - What does my care plan look like over a longer period of time?
    - Over time, will care providers come to me or will I need to make arrangements to visit them?
- Prior to going home, will I have the opportunity to get assistance

regarding assessing changes that could be made in my home, thereby allowing me safer living and more ability for normal living? (It might be on a temporary or more permanent basis.)

- Extra stair railings, grab bars in the bathroom, towel bars in higher or lower locations
- Removal of small rugs to prevent tripping, or additional chairs in which to rest when crossing a large room
- Tools to assist in dressing, reaching objects
- Providing access to all I need if using stairs is not possible while living in a two-story house with bedroom and main bathroom upstairs

• When does the doctor anticipate I will be able to resume normal activities like driving, hiking or long walks, cooking, lifting anything more than a few pounds? Add your questions based on your lifestyle and situation:

-
-
-
-
-

• What do I need to do to meet the doctor's anticipated time-frames?

The reality check about what happens after going home

- What would I normally be doing?
  - All my housework
  - Grocery shopping
  - Bathing
  - Effect of restrictions of movement
- What are the expectations of my family, employer, etc.?
  - I'll be back to normal in a couple of weeks
  - Ready to go back to work soon
- What are my expectations of myself?
  - I'll be good as new, or I'll never be OK again
  - If I do everything the doctor says, the sky's the limit
- How am I communicating to others what I can actually do now?
  - Sharing my doctor's plan and prognosis with family and others
  - Stating clearly what I can do
  - Asking directly what others' expectations are for me
- Do I know and can I communicate to others how my healing and progress will go?
- Do I need help figuring this out and if so, who can assist me?

When you come to a fork in the road, take it.
—Yogi Berra

CHAPTER 10

OTHER RESOURCES

～

*A*dding to the already extensive list of questions, the following are ones about where and how to find people, options, or equipment needed. The solution to many of these issues depends on whether your insurance covers the expenses and services you need or whether you have to find a more creative solution.

Equipment for self-care or rehabilitation

This category includes tools to pull your socks or pants up, additions to raise your toilet height allowing you to sit without using all your stomach muscles to get up and down, hospital beds, crutches, canes, and an incredibly long list of other items.

With insurance

Contact your assigned case manager, the assigned representative, the Q&A at the insurance website, or your company's human resources department. Ideally, you will get what you need directly from your insurance company. They won't want to know your whole history, just the claim #, your policy #, and the questions you have.

Be sure you are clear on what it will pay and which vendors you must use. Ask if the insurance rep, the doctor's office, or you are responsible and authorized to place the order or request. Be sure to get the doctor's request or authorization when insurance requires it. When your insurance company says it won't pay for something your doctor orders, find out if it is covered in your policy but called something else. If it goes by another name or category, your doctor could order it as the insurance notes it.

If your situation wasn't an accident, you have had time to know whom to contact and get at least some of the authorizations in place. For example, I knew I would need some self-care equipment after I left rehab and went home. At rehab I got expert recommendations and got approval from the doctor, whose office contacted my insurance caseworker. That allowed the insurance company to order the equipment, since it was the necessary process for those costs to be covered. It also ensured the equipment would be delivered to my home as I needed it.

Without insurance

You may have no insurance or insurance that covers the surgery but not all durable goods, which is another name for some equipment you may need so you can be at home rather than in a care facility. Here is a list of some ways you might get the equipment you need. Be sure, however you get your needs met, that the equipment actually works and someone who knows the equipment and your needs can help set it up and train you to use it properly.

Add your own creative ideas

- Ask your doctor, office staff, or any medical providers you are seeing if they have recommendations on where to get the equipment free or inexpensively.
- Check on an Internet site such as craigslist.
- Check garage and estate sales.

- Check at Goodwill, Salvation Army, or other service-related stores.
- Ask friends, friends of friends, in person, Facebook, Twitter, your workplace bulletin board, if allowed, to see if anyone has what you need. You might be surprised how many people have equipment from prior experiences in their attics or garages.
- Go online or directly to stores and see if they have discontinued items for rent for short periods of time.

Nursing care, personal care, physical therapy, and occupational therapy

I hope you have had the opportunity to talk to your doctor about what to expect after surgery, which will allow you and all who will be assisting you to have realistic expectations of whether you need to go to an interim care facility or can go directly home. This will give you an idea of what your initial needs and care might be like in either situation. If you are going through your insurance company, you may need preapprovals via doctor orders for use at certain facilities or caregivers. If you don't have insurance, be sure your doctor knows and can help you get the best care possible for what you can afford. You'll need a real conversation with your doctor about showing a family member how to assist when that is feasible, the minimum amount of professional care needed, and any care you need that can be done well in the most realistic cost-cutting manner.

Remember, hospitals and medical providers want you to get healthy and back to your most normal living possible. Many have extra services and ideas to help you find the best follow-up care and information regardless of your financial situation. Be respectful and honest in your requests, and usually you will be met with the same.

- What is your situation?
- What will you need help with (no detail is too small to consider)? A starting list could include assistance getting showered, hair washed, food preparation, laundry.

- What professional services will you really need? You might need physical therapy or a nurse to change bandages. If you don't have insurance, ask for assistance in sorting out what family members or friends could do safely and if any training is available to them.

What to do about pain

This topic requires an honest conversation with your doctor prior to surgery. Any allergic reactions to drugs should be in your file. If you have had any dependency issues, tell your doctor so that your risk for further problems in that area can be minimized. If you never had surgery or used any of the typical drugs used post op, be prepared for more pain at first than you had imagined. Don't be a hero about not taking the medications, but let your doctor know you want to get off narcotic pain relief as soon as possible. Aside from possible addiction, major constipation is often a side effect. If you don't have insurance, ask your doctor to prescribe generic medications whenever the results will be as effective as brand-name drugs.

Even if the surgery is successful, you may still be left with pain, sometimes significant pain. Keep an open mind. Talk to your doctor and with others who live with pain and have found some relief. I suggest that drugs should be used sparingly or as a last resort. Here are some options as well as ideas for getting information:

- Look online for pain relief specific to your situation, but beware. Remember that the Internet is full of both helpful truths and as many scams.
- Check for online communities, blogs, or chats specific to your situation. If you can't find one, start one.
- Be open minded about trying meditation, acupuncture, and other widely accepted nontraditional approaches.
- Develop a sense of new normal, in which the idea that you must be completely pain free can be replaced by a desire to live as pain free as is realistically possible.

- Check with your doctor and physical and occupational therapists about the latest treatments available. New products and procedures are being introduced all the time.
- Investigate with a pain physician regarding a treatment plan for chronic pain. Consider the scope from conservative to aggressive.

Whether you have opted not to have surgery or had surgery that didn't relieve all your pain, stay hopeful. There are many ways that life can have meaning. Sometimes it involves a new lifestyle, viewpoint, or solution never considered. Here are a few examples of what might be available.

- This solution would probably be offered in the pain doctor's office, or you might find it online and ask your doctor about it. It doesn't cure pain, but for those who find it effective, real pain reduction is the result. It is neurostimulation, also known as spinal cord stimulation. First, your doctor would do an assessment to see if you are a good candidate. Then a test period of the procedure would be done that involves temporarily implanting thin wires. There is also an external programmer. In simplistic terms, the device takes the pain and rather than sending that message to the brain, replaces it with a different sensation. The sensations can range from a mild massaging feeling to no sensation at all. It doesn't take long to determine whether this plan works. If it does, surgery and more complete implantation are done. There is, of course, much more to this, but I mention the process only to give an idea of the variety of solutions that may be available.
- Physical therapy management of pain can introduce new ways of moving and being active. Specialists will work with you and your doctor to determine the exact source of your pain and how it impacts your body as well as the best way to relieve it as you go through your daily living. If you have had surgery, they will help you determine realistic timeframes for easing back into normal

activities. They will work with you to look at every aspect of your daily living and goals to find creative ways of enhancing your abilities. You have to do your part, too, which may mean exercises, changing old behaviors, and being open to change.

- Home assistance agencies assist with everyday activities as well as with medical needs. Many are based on an hourly fee, and their people are trained and bonded. Be open to receive extra help in the areas that are most difficult for you. For instance, if you can't perform an activity around the house or need assistance with shopping, get help for that. Being restored or living normally is not an all-or-nothing proposition.
- Become knowledgeable about your medical situation. Attend lectures at a teaching hospital, read articles, connect with others in your situation, and learn what realistic expectations are and what relief is available to you. Don't believe that nothing more can be done for you without getting second and third opinions.

This resource section is only a slice of the needs and plans involved in any major medical difficulty. Especially pertinent to the United States, it is general in nature because there is such a large range of options, determined in part by the state you live in, your age, and your personal resources. Regardless of where assistance will come from, the needs are real. My hope is that these resources facilitate a positive dialogue among family members, the medical team, and all concerned parties.

*When one door of happiness closes, another one opens;
but often we look so long at the closed door that we do
not see the one which has opened for us.*
—Helen Keller

TODAY

I hope *My Life as a Metal Sculpture* has been useful. I've shared where I started from, how I moved forward, the impact on others, and their insights as well as resources you can use. If you have read and will use anything from this book, you share my desire to make the best of life as is possible.

Something else we have in common is the action we can take today only. We can reflect and learn from the past and make plans for the future, but today is the day of action.

I would love to hear from you on my blog site:

mylifeasametalsculpture.blogspot.com

This will also be a good way to learn about events and projects associated with the book.

The blog has more details from others' perspectives and new information as well as details of my story. You also have the opportunity to share experiences you think might benefit other readers.

I would also like to know if you would like a similar book more specific to other types of medical trauma, like heart conditions, cancer, or a more specific injury. Is there something in the book you would like more detail about, or did you expect some type of information that wasn't covered well? Would workbooks and workshops to personalize the resources section be helpful?

Today you can seek the balance unique just to you. Remember, even in the midst of serious subjects and serious times, don't underestimate the healing and balancing power of humor. There is nothing like a spontaneous smile or heartfelt laugh to instantly restore perspective. There are online sites devoted to quotes of all sorts from spiritual to humorous, as well as great options at your local bookstore. One book I recommend is *The Yogi Book* (Workman, NY: 1999, 2010) by Yogi Berra, which includes his smile-producing comments as well as his recollections.

Carol R. Palo

Acknowledgements

*I*n the spirit of deep appreciation. . .

To write about personal events and share that journey are big decisions, especially true if you are not an author by trade but rather are moved to help others by using your experiences. Without the following people, my story would be less helpful, and my desire to detail how to best navigate through medical adversity would be less thorough. Thank you to the friends who stood by me during the process of pain, surgery, and recovery, especially those who shared their insights and experiences in this book. There aren't adequate words to express the importance of my family for courage, loyalty, and love. I am still moved by thoughts of my daughter stepping in for anything that needed to be done and my son's willingness to quit a job he loved to take care of me, if necessary. In addition, without the support of brave acquaintances and friends who were willing to read the early drafts, provide technical information, and offer honest feedback, the task might have been too daunting.

I'm not a person who looked for heroes in my life, but as a result of this medical adversity, the doctor who first spotted my spinal problems and the surgeon who provided the solution are my heroes today. In addition, a good friend, Linda Faino, shared this with me:

> People are like stained glass windows—
> the true beauty can be seen only when
> there is light from within. The darker the night,
> the brighter the windows.
>
> —Elisabeth Kubler-Ross

Linda showed me how it is possible not only to quote words of beauty but also how to live them. In the same category are the Luber and Stier families as well as Bill Wilson and Dr. Bob Smith for their program of hope, and my parents for their unconditional love.

After my surgery and recovery, I was approached by many people who had never had to face the consequences of a serious medical adversity and didn't know best how to deal with the medical community, make plans, and find resources. I appreciate these people reaching out because their actions also convinced me of the need to detail my journey.

I want to thank the Willamette Writers Annual Conference, where I received my first encouraging, realistic look at what needs to be done after the book is written. Very exciting to me is membership in the Northwest Writers and Publishers Association, which provides a nurturing mix of writers, editors, film and other media people, and monthly programs that have given me what I needed as each next step came up. I can't imagine producing an understandable book without the assistance of copy editor Sue Mann of Working With Words, Emily Goetz's creative illustration of my spine, photography by Hugh Penland, and the guiding hand of Luminare Press.

CPSIA information can be obtained at www.ICGtesting.com
Printed in the USA
BVOW07s1636131113

336177BV00002B/8/P